Face Reading

Self-Care and Natural Healing
through **Traditional Chinese Medicine**

By Wu Jianshe

SCPG

This book is edited and designed by the Editorial Committee of *Cultural China* series.

Text by Wu Jianshe
Translation by Wu Yanting
Design by Wang Wei

Copy Editor: Shelly Bryant
Editor: Cao Yue
Editorial Director: Zhang Yicong

ISBN: 978-1-93836-859-2

Address any comments about *Face Reading: Self-Care and Natural Healing through Traditional Chinese Medicine* to:

SCPG
401 Broadway, Ste.1000
New York, NY 10013
USA

or

Shanghai Press and Publishing Development Co., Ltd.
390 Fuzhou Road, Shanghai, China (200001)
Email: sppdbook@163.com
Printed in China by Shanghai Donnelley Printing Co., Ltd.

1   3   5   7   9   10   8   6   4   2

The material in this book is provided for informational purposes only and is not intended as medical advice. The information contained in this book should not be used to diagnose or treat any illness, disorder, disease or health problem. Always consult your physician or health care provider before beginning any treatment of any illness, disorder or injury. Use of this book, advice, and information contained in this book is at the sole choice and risk of the reader.

Contents

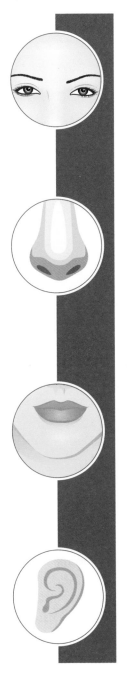

Introduction

According to traditional Chinese medicine (TCM), "You know the ailment when you see a person's face, which is divine." In fact, most diseases leave traces that can be detected on the surface of the human body where the twelve principal meridians[1] and the Governor and Conception vessels that connect the internal organs run. That is why it is often said that "the symptoms are manifested in the four limbs and five sensory organs, while the diseases are deep in the five viscera organs (*zang*) and six bowels (*fu*)."

With a long history in China, face reading in TCM is based on thousands of years of valuable experience accumulated from generations of Chinese medical practitioners. The five sensory organs in the face are not only some of the important human organs, but they are also where the meridian pathways run,

---

1 Meridian. In the TCM theoretical system, a meridian is considered a system that communicates between the exterior and interior of the human body and connects with the five *zang* and six *fu* organs inside the body. These meridians, which run across the body vertically, linking the interior with the exterior and the top with the bottom part of the body, and the internal organs, extremities, and joints, are responsible for carrying and distributing *qi* and blood to nourish the muscles and bones. There are roughly twelve principal meridians, which include the Taiyin Lung Meridian of the Hand, the Jueyin Pericardium Meridian of the Hand, the Shaoyin Heart Meridian of the Hand, the Yangming Large Intestine Meridian of the Hand, the Shaoyang *Sanjiao* Meridian of the Hand, the Taiyang Small Intestine Meridian of the Hand, the Yangming Stomach Meridian of the Foot, the Shaoyang Gallbladder Meridian of the Foot, the Taiyang Bladder Meridian of the Foot, the Taiyin Spleen Meridian of the Foot, the Jueyin Liver Meridian of the Foot, and the Shaoyin Kidney Meridian of the Foot, along with the Governor Vessels and the Conception Vessel.

connecting the *zang* and *fu* organs[1] inside the human body. By observing the face, a doctor can detect changes in *zang-fu, qi*[2] and blood, muscles and bones, meridians and collaterals[3], and essential *qi*, thereby gathering information to make judgments on the causes of a disease, establish the pathogenesis, predict the tendency of the disease and sequela, and determine the prognosis. Such information plays a crucial role in the treatment of an ailment.

Guided by the theories of traditional Chinese medicine, face reading not only helps diagnose diseases but has also become increasingly popular for prognosis and maintaining good health. The methods it utilizes are unique and produce effective results. Both economical and safe, face reading is easy to learn and use, making it an ideal means of daily healthcare.

With the aim of disseminating the knowledge of TCM, this book first introduces the fundamentals of face reading in a systematic, scientific manner, then offers a detailed explanation of the methods used to detect many common ailments. Given the capacity of each disease's natural self-healing power, also provided here are physiotherapeutic treatment and internal adjustment measures, such as dietary remedies, physical exercises, and emotional adjustments. Through rich content and a combination of graphics and texts that are easy to understand, this book is a practical, popular primer that even people having no knowledge of traditional Chinese medicine can understand and use for self-diagnosis and self-treatment.

Chapter One
Understanding Face Reading

Whether a person is healthy or not can be ascertained by observing the face and sensory organs. In TCM, the human face is considered the external representations of the viscera, *qi*, and blood. It is also where the meridians gather, and therefore the prosperity and decline of the *zang* and *fu* organs and the disturbance of vital *qi* and blood by evil *qi* will be reflected in the face. For example, a healthy person's face glows, looking attractive and moist, meaning that person has sufficient nourishing *qi* and blood. If a person's face looks dull or bloodless, it may suggest problems with that person's internal organs. Therefore, face reading plays a crucial role in diagnostic inspection in traditional Chinese medicine. By observing the face, a doctor can perceive the changes happening within the viscera, *qi* and blood, muscles, joints and bones, meridians, and

---

1 *Zang* and *fu* organs. The general term for the internal organs of the human body. It is mainly divided into five *zang* organs and six *fu* organs. The five *zang* organs are the heart, the liver, the spleen, the lung, and the kidney. The six *fu* organs are the gallbladder, the stomach, the large intestine, the small intestine, the bladder, and the triple burners.

2 *Qi*. The most fundamental and micro-substance that constitutes a human being and sustains all human activity. *Qi* also denotes the physiological functions of the human body. In TCM, it expresses different meanings when used in combination with other word(s).

3 Collaterals. In TCM there are the main trunks and branches that transport *qi* and blood in the human body. These passages are classified into meridians and collaterals, of which the main trunks running vertically are called meridians and the channels branching out from the main trunks are called collaterals.

the vital *qi*, thereby understanding the prosperity and decline of the vital *qi* and the depth of penetration of evil *qi*, thus predicting the course of pathological changes. This chapter focuses on the concept of face reading, its theoretical foundation, and the corresponding relationship between the sensory organs on the face and the internal organs, as well as some cautionary tips in conducting face reading. It explores the rich wisdom of face reading by following an experienced TCM doctor.

1. Basic Concepts

Face reading is one aspect of the diagnostic inspection of traditional Chinese medicine, a method through which a TCM doctor observes on a patient's face the reflex zones pertaining to the viscera organs and learns about the health conditions of that person's viscera. With an overview of the face and the sensory organs in mind, the doctor learns the functional states of the body's viscera, the meridians, and the *qi* and blood, thereby arriving at a conclusion about the general and localized pathological changes of the person's body. Put simply, one can "look at the sensory organs on the face and inspect the state of *qi* and blood, and the diseases of *zang* and *fu* organs can be determined."

Specifically, diagnostic face reading relies on the inspection of several things.

The color and brightness of the face. By observing the color and brightness of facial skin, a doctor determines the prosperity and decline of *qi* and blood and the progression of a pathological development, thereby predicting a person's health conditions. For example, the skin color of a Chinese person is yellow, and when the facial skin looks rosy with radiance, it is a healthy complexion. When it looks otherwise, it may indicate a health problem.

The shape and bearing of a person. There is much to be read in a person's physical shape and bearing. People who are overweight but actually eat very little are most likely to experience a spleen deficiency and phlegm retention, while those who are skinny but eat a lot often have excess stomach fire[1]. A person's bearing is a manifestation of that person's general state of health. People who are quiet and do not like to move much often experience cold syndromes[2]. People who are easily irritated and like to move a lot are most likely to have heat syndromes[3].

The general spirit. A person's spirit is the comprehensive manifestation of that person's vitality. Decisions are generally made through observing one's spirit, the look in one's eyes, the facial expression, their language ability, and their responsiveness. If a person has acute awareness, speaks clearly and is quick to respond, and the eyes look clear and bright, these are manifestations that the person is healthy. Conversely, if a person is often incoherent and has a dull look in the eyes, an apathetic facial expression, and slow responses, and also exhibits a general lassitude, it means that this person is in a state of sickness and may even be seriously ill.

The five sensory organs on the face. Inspecting the five

---

1 Stomach fire. A pathological development caused by exuberance of stomach heat turning into fire. Primary symptoms include heartburn and acid reflux, pain in the stomach, abdominal fullness, dry mouth and bad breath, swollen and painful gums, and constipation or loose stool. Stomach fire is also called stomach heat, and it is usually triggered by indulgence in alcohol or excessive intake of pungent, oily foods and poor dietary habits.

2 Cold syndrome. A syndrome characterized by the repression of the functional capacity of the human body due to the invasion of cold pathogens or hyperactivity of the *yin* leading to a *yang* deficiency. The syndromes are manifested as cold and chill.

3 Heat syndrome. A syndrome characterized by warm and heat features. It is the result of hyperactivity in the body due to an attack of heat pathogens, hyperactivity of the *yang* in the internal organs, or overactive *yang* due to a *yin* deficiency. Clinical manifestations are a feverish sensation, aversion to heat and preference for cold, constant desire for liquids due to thirst, redness in the face, irritability and anxiety, thick, yellow nasal discharge and sputum, scanty yellow urine, dry stool, and red tongue with little saliva.

sensory organs is an important aspect of face reading diagnosis. TCM teaches that the five viscera organs open to the five sensory organs and, therefore, one can learn the health conditions of the viscera through observing the five sensory organs on the face. The eyes are the orifices of the liver, and therefore diseases associated with the liver are often reflected in the eyes. For example, if the eyes are red and swollen, it is usually a result of liver fire[1] or wind-heat[2]. The kidneys open into the ears and, therefore, problems associated with the kidneys often manifest themselves in the ears. For example, if the pinna of the ear looks scorched black and withered, it is usually a sign of insufficient kidney essence[3]. The lungs open into the nose. If a pathogen develops in the lungs, the nose will perform abnormally, e.g. a twitching nose signifies pathogenic heat congesting lung[4].

    Tongue signs. Diagnosis through the tongue signs is a unique diagnostic procedure based on the experiences accumulated by TCM practices over time. It is conducted by looking at the texture of the tongue, i.e. the muscular part of the tongue, and the tongue coating, i.e. the moss-like covering on the tongue surface. Tongue texture can reveal the state of deficiency and excess of the viscera while the tongue coating can reveal the depth of external evil invasion of the body. A healthy person has a tongue that is pale red in color with a thin layer of white coating. Abnormalities of the tongue can be determined through its color and coating. For example, when the tongue is red, it signifies heat, and when pale white, it indicates deficiency and cold. A purple tongue suggests blood stasis, and a yellow one implies interior[5] and heat syndromes. When the tongue is white, it denotes superficies[6] and cold syndromes.

2. Theoretical Foundation

The human face is where meridians gather. By observing the face, one can acquire physiological information about various parts of the body. In addition, the facial skin, which is thin and located at the highest part of the human body, is more likely to manifest color changes, which are easier to detect in diagnostic inspection.

After extensive medical practices over a long period, traditional Chinese medicine has gradually come to the realization that the human body is an integrated organic whole, with the five *zang* organs at the center, the meridians serving as pathways, *qi* and blood serving as the media that connect the internal organs with the external skin, sensory organs, and four limbs of the body. All parts of the human body are interdependent and influence one another. Therefore, changes in the internal tissues and organs will be manifest in the external appearance of the body. Changes in the external appearance of the body will also affect the internal tissues and organs. Local

---

1 Liver fire. Exuberance of liver fire that exceeds the tolerance of the human body turns to a pathogenic fire. The causes are mostly emotional factors, improper dietary habits, and pathogenic fire transmitted to the liver meridian. The symptoms are manifested as lightheadedness, redness in the face and eyes, a bitter taste in the mouth, irritability or a short temper, constipation, and yellow urine.

2 Wind-heat. Pathogens of wind and heat simultaneously attack the human body to cause diseases. The clinical manifestations are high fever, mild chills, coughing, and thirst.

3 Essence. Essence is an umbrella term that encompasses all physical substances in the body, including *qi*, blood, body fluids, and nutrient essence.

4 Pathogenic heat congesting lung. Internal stagnation of pathogenic heat in the lungs, which often invades through the mouth and nose, or wind-cold and wind-heat invading the interior, thereby transforming the hyperactivity of *yang* into febrile diseases blocking the lung.

5 Interior syndrome. As opposed to superficies syndrome, interior syndrome indicates that the pathological changes have entered deep into the *zang* and *fu* organs, *qi*, blood, and bone marrow, such that the illness is in the internal part of the body and the condition is more severe and lingering.

6 Superficies syndrome. Pathological changes that occur in the superficial part of the body and are often regarded as in the early stage of a disease. Also called exterior syndrome.

pathological change can have an impact on the whole body. Conversely, systemic pathological changes can also reveal changes locally through such organs as eyes, nose, lips and ears. Therefore, by observing the changes in shape and color of these body parts on the face, the functional state of the internal organs can be roughly understood. This is the theoretical foundation on which face reading is based. In fact, a relatively exhaustive theoretical system was formed as early as the *Inner Canon of the Yellow Emperor* (*Huangdi Neijing*). As that classic puts it, "Look at the external appearance, and you know the internal organs, and

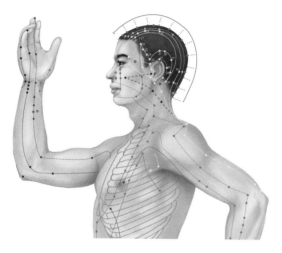

- - - - - Taiyin Lung Meridian of the Hand (LU)
————— Taiyin Spleen Meridian of the Foot (SP)
- - - - - Jueyin Pericardium Meridian of the Hand (PC)
————— Jueyin Liver Meridian of the Foot (LR)
- - - - - Shaoyin Heart Meridian of the Hand (HT)
- - - - - Taiyang Small Intestine Meridian of the Hand (SI)
————— Taiyang Bladder Meridian of the Foot (BL)
- - - - - Yangming Large Intestine Meridian of the Hand (LI)
————— Yangming Stomach Meridian of the Foot (ST)
- - - - - Shaoyang *Sanjiao*[1] Meridian of the Hand (TE)
————— Shaoyang Gallbladder Meridian of the Foot (GB)

Principal meridians of the human body.

thereby what the ailment is."

Although physical changes often take place gradually, which is a slow process that is hard to detect, there are always clues you can find. It is important, then, to keep an eye on the sensory organs on the face in order to detect the subtle changes that are taking place and discover the cause of the disease, which in turn will help prevent the onset of an illness and avoid the worsening of the disease.

In addition, the human face presents a collection of physiological information about various parts of the body, making it a microcosm of the whole human body. Different parts of the face pertain to different *zang* and *fu* organs, which is the basis of face reading diagnosis. The distribution of *zang* and *fu* organs on the face is derived from the theories stated in the *Inner Canon of the Yellow Emperor* of *zang xiang* (i.e., the internal organs and the manifestations of their physiological and pathological

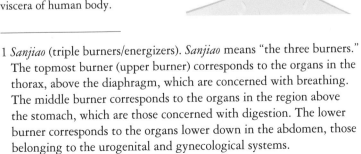

❶ Chest (Breast)	❾ Kidneys
❷ Head and face	❿ Small intestine
❸ Liver	⓫ Lower limbs
❹ Lungs	⓬ Stomach
❺ Gallbladder	⓭ Spleen
❻ Heart	⓮ Bladder
❼ Large intestine	⓯ Uterus
❽ Upper limbs	

Parts of the face pertaining to the viscera of human body.

---

1 *Sanjiao* (triple burners/energizers). *Sanjiao* means "the three burners." The topmost burner (upper burner) corresponds to the organs in the thorax, above the diaphragm, which are concerned with breathing. The middle burner corresponds to the organs in the region above the stomach, which are those concerned with digestion. The lower burner corresponds to the organs lower down in the abdomen, those belonging to the urogenital and gynecological systems.

states), *qi* and blood, and the distribution of meridians. For more details, see the picture on page 13.

If an abnormality occurs at a certain area of the face, it usually indicates that there is a problem with the internal organ pertaining to it. Please see the explanation below.

Mental stress zone: The upper third of the forehead to the hairline. If acne appears here, or if the skin color in this area is different from the general complexion of the face, it indicates that the person is experiencing mental stress. If skin spots occur, it means that pathogenic changes may have developed with the heart, e.g. cardiomyopathy. If a mole or wart develops, it points to a congenital problem with the function of the heart.

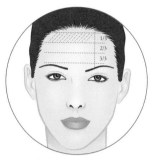

Mental stress zone.

Heart zone: On the bridge of the nose between the eyes. If horizontal creases develop or are clearly evident, it suggests arrhythmia or problematic heart conditions. If the horizontal creases here are deep, coupled with vertical cracks on the surface of the tongue, it often indicates a serious heart disease.

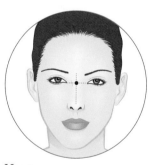

Heart zone.

Lung zone: The midpoint of the line linking the start of both eyes brows. If the forehead has a deeper than normal depression in the center or the skin color is dull or bluish, or there are skin spots, it means that the person is likely to have lung disease or breathing problems. If acne appears here, it suggests that the person may have had a cold or

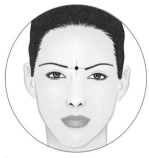

Lung zone.

sore throat recently. If there is a mole or wart at the start of the brow, or the skin color there is pale white, it indicates that this person may have laryngopharyngitis or tonsillitis, oppression in the chest and shortness of breath, or some kind of lung disease. If the part directly above the start of the brow bulges above the skin, it also suggests lung disease.

Chest (breast) zone: The area between the bridge of the nose and the inner corners of the eyes. If this part looks dull or bluish in a man, it suggests oppression in the chest and shortness of breath. If this part looks dull or bluish in a woman, it indicates that she may suffer from distending pain in the breast during menstruation. If there are moles or warts on the inner side of the upper eyelid or acne types of growth on the eyelid, it may indicate lobular hyperplasia in a woman or pleurisy in a man. If there are bumps in the inner corner of the eye, it reveals that she may have breast hyperplasia.

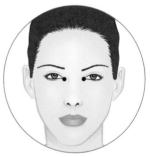

Chest (breast) zone.

Liver zone: The middle part (also the highest point) of the bridge of the nose. If this part appears bluish dark or develops skin spots, it suggests problems with the liver. If there is acne, it is a sign that this person has hyperactivity of the liver fire. If the higher part of the bridge of the nose has skin spots, it may mean hyperactivity of the liver fire[1]

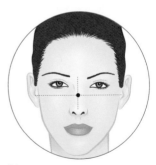

Liver zone.

---

1 Hyperactivity of the liver fire. A heat-related syndrome due to the hyperactivity of the liver function. It is most related to emotional factors, diet, and heat pathogens in other *zang-fu* organs affecting the liver meridian. Main clinical symptoms are lightheadedness, redness in the face and eyes, bitter taste in the mouth, and irritability and a short temper.

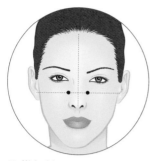

Gallbladder zone.

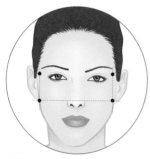

Kidney zone.

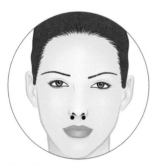

Bladder zone.

and an unbalanced emotional state. If the bluish skin color on the bridge of the nose reaches the tip of the nose, it is a warning sign of cancer or a tumor.

Gallbladder zone: The lateral surfaces straddling the higher part of the bridge of the nose. If this part shows blood streaks or acne, or if the mouth tastes bitter when getting up in the morning, it may suggest slight inflammation of the gallbladder. If there are skin spots, it points to cholecystitis. If there are vertical wrinkles, or vertical wrinkles appear when smiling, it suggests problems with the gallbladder. If there are moles or warts, the person may suffer from congenital functional deficiency of the gallbladder or gallstones.

Kidney zone: Directly beneath the temples to the line linking both ear lobes. If this part has blood streaks, acne or skin spots, it means that the person has a kidney deficiency or is manifesting tiredness, soreness, and pain of the back or lower back. If large, deep skin spots appear here, the person is likely to have kidney stones. If there are moles or warts, it suggests that the person suffers from a congenital deficiency of the kidney function and is manifesting soreness and pain in the back, lower back, and legs.

Bladder zone: The base of nose on both sides of the philtrum. If this part is red or has blood streaks, acne, abscesses, or other imperfections, it means that the person has a bladder inflammation. Associated symptoms are brownish urine, frequent urination, and soreness or pain in the lower back. When a woman has bladder inflammation, it is usually caused by gynaecological issues. However, if the base of the nose looks red, but there is no symptom of frequent urination or urgency of urination, coupled with the redness of the whole bridge of the nose, this may point to rhinitis.

Spleen zone: The nasal tip. If this part is reddish or swollen, or the person has rhinophyma, these are signs of spleen heat or the swelling of the spleen. Associated symptoms are heavy-headedness, aching cheeks and irritability. If the nasal tip looks yellowish or pale, it points to the deficiency of the spleen, manifesting symptoms such as profuse sweat, aversion to wind, weariness of the limbs, fatigue and loss of appetite.

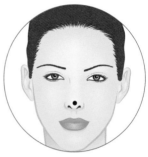

Spleen zone.

Stomach zone: The sides of the nostrils. If these appear reddish, it suggests stomach fire, manifesting in such symptoms as excessive hunger and bad breath. If blood streaks become pervasive, it warns of the possibility of gastritis. If they look bluish gray, it indicates stomach coldness. If they appear blue and withered, accompanied by a constant, prolonged stomachache, it means the person has atrophic gastritis. If the sides of the nostrils are thin with deep furrows, it could suggest atrophic gastritis.

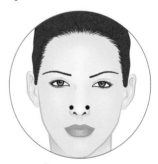

Stomach zone.

Small intestine zone: Beneath

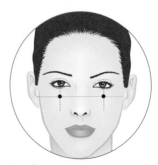

Small intestine zone.

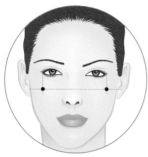

Large intestine zone.

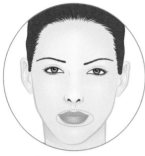

Reproductive system zone.

the cheekbones on the medial side. If this part has red streaks, acne, skin spots, moles, or warts, it indicates poor small intestinal absorption, causing the person to look physically thin and weak.

Large intestine zone: Beneath the cheekbones on the lateral side. If this part has blood streaks, acne, skin spots, moles, or warts, it is an indication of defecation dysfunctions of the large intestine, and the person tends to experience dry stool, constipation, or loose stool. If this part has crescent-shaped skin spots, it means the person is susceptible to constipation or has haemorrhoids.

Reproductive system zone: The philtrum and around the lips. If a female has moles or warts below the lips and her chin looks reddish but the kidney zone is smooth and clean, it usually indicates that this person experiences soreness and pain in the lower back. If a female has moles or warts around her lips, or the area surrounding her lips appears bluish, black or pale, accompanied by abnormalities in the kidney zone, it often means that person is frigid. If a woman has a mole in the philtrum, it points to problems with the uterus. If a man has moles or warts above his lips, with abnormalities in the kidney zone, it suggests problems with his reproductive system. If a male in his 40s and above has a thicker upper lip, that means he may have enlarged prostate. If he has recurrent acne on his lips, it means that he has prostatitis. A man whose upper lip is not smooth and has furrows on it may have problems of sexual dysfunction.

3. Cautions

Face reading is best done in the morning. It is best to check your face in the morning when your *qi* and blood status is neither disturbed nor affected by other factors such as mood changes and exercise. In the morning, your complexion is most natural, and therefore it is easy to detect disease through facial inspection. With a good understanding of the changes in your complexion, you will find signs of any ailment that is developing in your body in a timely manner.

Do not wear makeup for face reading. Cosmetics conceal the true color of your facial skin, which is not conducive to disease detection. For example, a sallow complexion is a manifestation of a spleen deficiency syndrome[1], but a ruddy complexion due to facial makeup may lead the doctor to a wrong diagnosis. Wearing lipstick can make a person with pale lips, a sign of *yang* deficiency[2], appear "normal" or with balanced *qi* and blood. Therefore, patients are advised against wearing makeup before seeing their doctor. Let the doctor see you in your most natural state for an accurate diagnosis.

Do not consume colored foods or drinks before face reading. Before a face reading session, the consumption of certain foods or drugs with color, such as tomatoes, licorice

---

1 Deficiency syndrome. Deficiency of vital *qi* resulting in reduced body resistance to diseases and impaired functioning of the physical body. Manifestations are pale complexion and pale colored lips, tiredness and fatigue, general malaise, shortness of breath, palpitations, spontaneous sweats and night sweats, loose stool, and frequent urination.

2 *Yang* deficiency. The insufficiency of *yang* leading to the decline of the body's warming function, which brings about a series of clinical symptoms that are mostly developed from long-term *qi* deficiency. It is also associated with dietary habits, living in a cold residence for a long time, long-term illness of the elderly, and congenital weakness in the physical constitution.

tablets, or black plums, may lead to misdiagnosis, because tomato will turn your mouth cavity and lips reddish, while food such as black plums tend to make the tongue coating black. Coffee, egg yolks, oranges, yellow pills, and oral liquids will make the tongue coating look yellow. All these affect the color of the face and tongue coating, and thereby can lead to misdiagnosis.

Stay calm and relaxed during face reading. A person's state of mind is also a factor for consideration. When people are angry, sad, or in a state of ecstasy, their complexion will turn a different color than usual. Therefore, maintain peace of mind and body during face reading so your complexion will not be affected by these emotional factors.

Seasonal changes affect complexion. Human complexion changes as the seasons change. In spring the complexion is faintly greenish, slightly red in summer but pale yellowish in prolonged summer (i.e., the last eighteen days of each season), pale in fall, and a bit dark in winter.

Chapter Two
Face Reading Methods

This chapter discusses the methods of conducting facial reading by inspecting the face as a whole, then moving onto the individual parts, such as the eyes, ears, nose, lips, tongue, and teeth. The *Lingshu (Spiritual Pivot)* from the traditional Chinese medicine classic the *Inner Canon of the Yellow Emperor* says, "The *qi* and blood of twelve meridians and 365 channels all ascend to the face and its orifices." Rich with the collaterals and nourished by exuberant *qi* and blood, the face's tender, thin skin is more revealing as far as color changes are concerned. In addition, the *zang* and *fu* organs of the human body are also represented in the corresponding areas of the face and sense organs. Therefore, closely watching the changes in the color and shape of the facial features can effectively help you make a judgment on your own state of health.

1. General Diagnosis of the Face

There are two aspects to observe when conducting face reading, the color radiance and physical form.

Complexion is likened to a thermometer that helps one understand his or her health status. By observing the changes in the color and radiance of one's facial skin, one can tell whether the *zang* and *fu* organs are in a state of deficiency or excess, the *qi* and blood are prosperous or on the decline, the nature of the disease is a cold or heat type, and the severity of the disease and its prognosis. All of these combined can lead to a conclusion about whether a person is healthy.

Diagnosis through inspecting the complexion is mainly carried out by observing the changes in the color and radiance of the facial skin. When looking at a person's complexion, it is important to compare the color during illness with its normal color and compare the patient's skin color with that of a group of people's to arrive at a judgment. Second, observe the change in the radiance of the skin color. When a change occurs in the pathological development, the radiance of the facial skin changes. Third, judgment should be primarily based on the general complexion of the patient, but its radiance and moistness or dullness constitute the key basis for judgment. In addition, face reading should not be confounded by factors unrelated to diseases, e.g. no face reading should be conducted right after physical exercise.

There are mainly four types of complexions.

Red complexion. When the facial skin is red, it generally indicates that there is heat in the body. *Qi* and blood flow smoothly when they are warm. When heat is abundant and blood vessels are full, the color of the blood is reflected in the skin, making the face red.

When accompanied by a red, swelling, and sore throat, it indicates an exogenous wind-heat attack, i.e. wind and heat combined invading the human body.

A very red edge of the face indicates heat in the Yangming meridian, one of the twelve principal meridians of the human body. Heat in the Yangming meridian refers to the exuberance of heat pathogens pervading the Yangming meridian.

When accompanied by insomnia or irritability with hot sensation in the chest, palms, and soles, it indicates endogenous heat[1] due to *yin* deficiency[2]. *Yin* is only deficient when compared with a normal state of *yang*, because when *yin* (cold in property) is insufficient, *yang* (hot in property) becomes excess as a result, and a general relative heat condition is established.

A pale complexion with redness in cheekbones, accompanied by shortness of breath, limbs cold up to the elbows and

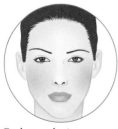

Red complexion.

knees indicates long-term illness leading to *yang* deficiency and *yin* exuberance, i.e. excess of internal *yin* leading to damage of *yang*.

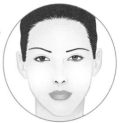

White complexion. When a person's complexion lacks the color of blood, this person is considered to have a "white complexion" because the lack of blood results in the failure of nutritive blood to nourish the face. White mainly indicates a deficient cold syndrome[3] and a syndrome of blood deficiency[4], which are the result of the deficiency of both *qi* and blood, leading to a failed nourishment of the body.

White complexion.

Pale complexion, weight loss, and lightheadedness indicate an internal blood deficiency, i.e. there is not sufficient amount

---

1 Endogenous heat. Also called internal fire. In TCM theory, it is considered fire or heat that originates internally. It is a general manifestation of the imbalance of *yin* and *yang* in the human body due to various factors. It is often associated with the invasion of exogenous pathogenic *qi*, an imbalanced diet, emotional factors, prolonged illness, and overactive sexual activity.

2 *Yin* deficiency. Deficiency of *yin* fluid leads to the decline of its function to moisturize and calm and its potential to averse descension, formation, and counterbalance *yang* and heat. As a result, deficient heat syndrome occurs as characterized by relatively hyperactive *yang* symptoms such as dryness, heat, ascension, agitation, and excessive vaporization. Deficiency of *yin* fluid can lead to deficiency heat occurring internally.

3 Deficient cold syndrome. This syndrome refers to *yang* deficiency due to exuberance of *yin* cold in the interior, which cannot replenish *zang-fu* organs. Often seen in ailments such as edema, diarrhea, palpitation, stomachache, and delayed menstruation.

4 Blood deficiency. Insufficiency of blood leading to failure to either nourish *zang-fu* organ, meridians, collaterals, or the physical body or to sustain the normal spiritual activities of a human. This is mainly caused by congenital weaknesses in the physical constitution, long-term illness, anxiety or worry, weaknesses of the spleen and stomach, and excessive blood loss.

of blood in the body to fully nourish *zang* and *fu* organs, the meridians and collaterals, and the physical shape, nor can it sustain the normal mental activity of a human being.

Dullness in the complexion and general malaise indicate the decline of *yang*.

A pale complexion and severe abdominal pain indicate internal hyperactivity of cold, i.e. pathogenic cold invading the body and damaging *yang*, which leads to the retention of pathogenic cold in the body.

Pale complexion, profuse perspiration but feeling cold, and limbs cold up to the elbows and knees indicate a sudden depletion of *yang* in the body.

Yellow complexion. Yellow is a reflection of a damp stagnancy due to a spleen deficiency. When the spleen, which rules transformation and transportation, experiences dysfunction in transportation, water and dampness cannot be vaporized, and when the spleen fails in its function of transformation due to a spleen deficiency, nutrient essence cannot be transformed into the *qi* and blood to nourish the skin, turning the skin yellow.

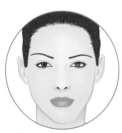

Yellow complexion.

A pale yellow complexion and haggard look indicates a spleen and stomach *qi* deficiency[1].

Yellow complexion and puffiness indicate a dysfunction of the spleen in transportation[2], resulting in the retention of pathogenous dampness in the body.

An orange-yellow complexion indicates retention of damp-heat[3] in the body.

A yellow complexion with a smoky dark tinge indicate a cold-dampness obstruction, i.e. cold-dampness[4] stagnation obstructing the flow of blood.

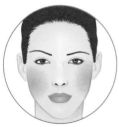

Black complexion.

Black complexion. Black is the color of the hyperactivity of water and exuberance of *yin*-cold. Deficiency and decline of kidney *yang*[5] results in fluid retention syndrome[6] leading to failure in water vaporization and

---

1 *Qi* deficiency. A pathological change due to exertion, fatigue, or deficiency of vital *qi* after severe or long-term illness, which leads to hypofunction of the *zang-fu* organ and tissue and reduced resistance to illness.

2 Dysfunction of the spleen in transportation. Damage of the spleen and stomach causing the dysfunction of spleen's capacity of transformation and transportation. Common symptoms are loss of appetite, abdominal fullness, particularly after a meal, loose stool, prolonged emaciation, sallow complexion, and general malaise.

3 Damp-heat. Both dampness and heat are pathogenic factors. They are two of the six evils/pathogens, which include wind, cold, summer heat, dampness, dryness, and fire (heat). Damp-heat usually refers to the syndrome of damp-heat, in which dampness and heat stagnate in the body obstructing the functions of *zang-fu* organ and meridians, resulting in pathological changes throughout the whole body featuring symptoms related to dampness and heat. This is often related to invasion of external pathogen, an improper diet, dysfunction of the spleen and stomach, and emotional factors. The symptoms are mainly tiredness and heaviness of the head and body, loss of appetite, abdominal fullness, nausea, a bitter taste in the mouth, difficulty emptying the bowels, loose stool, scanty urination that is yellow in color and foul in smell, and skin that is itchy, festering and oozing.

4 Cold-dampness. The invasion of a cold-damp pathogen or the retention of water due to deficiency of the spleen *yang*. This often occurs when one is caught in the rain and is affected by damp weather, when one sits or lies on a wet floor or ground, or when one eats cold, raw food. Clinical manifestations include heaviness in the head and body, painful joints and inflexibility of motion, lack of perspiration, weariness and aversion to cold, or facial puffiness and a swelling body that is worse in the low back and lower extremities, epigastric pain, loose stools, and difficulty urinating.

5 Kidney *yang*. In contrast to kidney *yin*, kidney *yang* warms, propels, moves, excites, and vaporizes.

6 Fluid retention syndrome. In TCM, *shui* (water in English) and *yin* (fluid) constitute a compound word, with each character holding equal importance. What is loose and clear is "water," e.g. sweat, urine. What is loose and sticky is "fluid," e.g. phlegm, nasal discharge. When abnormalities occur with regard to water and fluid in the body, fluid retention occurs.

qi transformation. Therefore, *yin* and cold prevails in the body, leading to failure of blood's function to nourish, the contraction of the limbs' tissue and tendons, and the inflexibility of limbs. This poor circulation of *qi* and blood leads to the blackening of the complexion as a result.

A black complexion with a yellow tinge that is dull and lusterless indicates deficiency of kidney *yang*, clinically characterized as "cold," with symptoms such as aversion to cold and cold limbs or soreness and aching of the lower back and knees.

A burnt black complexion with dryness, loss of head hair and shaky teeth indicates an overconsumption of kidney essence. This is often related to a congenital insufficiency, prolonged illness, or excessive sexual activity.

Dark rings surrounding the eyes indicate water diffusion due to kidney deficiency[1]. Deficiency of kidney essence and kidney *yang* results in failure in *qi* transformation[2], leading to diffusion of water in the body. The most common symptoms are edema, in the lower extremities in particular, scanty urine, tinnitus, and sore and weakened lower back and knees.

A black complexion, rough skin, and thirst with no desire to drink indicate a cold obstruction leading to stasis, i.e. pathogenic cold attacks the body, resulting in the obstruction of *yang*. The symptoms are severe chills, no perspiration, and pain in the head and body or chest and abdomen.

In addition to observing the facial complexion, physical changes in the face also reveal the health status of the interior of the human body. If the face lacks radiance and moisture and the skin is rough with many spots, this generally originates from the dysfunction of the five *zang* organs.

Puffiness of the face. This type of puffiness is caused by the obstruction of blood circulation due to the retention of too much water in the face. Usually one of the symptoms of some chronic diseases, puffiness of the face includes both emphysema and edema. The former is due to *qi* deficiency and the latter to water retention. Edema is more problematic than emphysema, and it requires more attention.

Puffiness, pale complexion, and shortness of breath indicate a deficiency of lung qi[3]. Symptoms include feeble, weak coughing, shortness of breath and panting that worsens with movement, clear, watery sputum, a low voice, spontaneous sweats, aversion to wind, and a pale tongue texture.

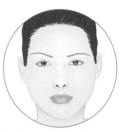

Puffiness of the face.

Localized swelling in the face indicates a deficiency of spleen *yang*. Deficiency and decline of spleen *yang* leads to the failure of the spleen's warming and transportation function. Common symptoms include fullness of the stomach even when not eating much, abdominal pain with a preference for warmth and pressure, aversion to cold and cold limbs, loose stool, edema in the lower limbs, or increased vaginal discharge in women.

Localized red swelling on the face is often the result of an allergy.

---

1 Water diffusion due to kidney deficiency. Deficiency of the kidney essence and kidney *yang* leading to failure in *qi* transformation and retention of water in the body. Symptoms are edema that is mostly evident in the lower limbs, scanty urine, tinnitus, aching and limp lower back and knees, pale tongue, and a white watery tongue coating.

2 Failure in *qi* transformation. *Qi* transformation is unable to be fulfilled due to deficiency of *yang qi*. This impairs the production and transformation of *qi*, blood, essence, and fluid, and as a result the elimination of metabolic products from fluid is obstructed and the retention of such metabolic products results in pathological changes in the body.

3 Deficiency of lung *qi*. Characterized by symptoms such as the weakening of lung *qi*, weak coughing, shortness of breath, and panting that worsens with activity, clear light phlegm, a low voice, or spontaneous perspiration and aversion to wind.

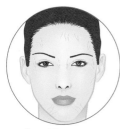

Evident blue veins on the face.

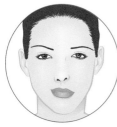

Face twitching.

A bloated face and body may suggest diseases of the kidneys or the heart.

Evident blue veins on the face. Blue veins appearing on the face usually mean stagnation of phlegm and dampness, stasis, and toxins in the body that are unable to be excreted, thereby obstructing the circulation of blood and *qi*, resulting in blue veins enlarged, dilated, twisted, and a change in color.

Bulging vein on the temples are a sign of dizziness and headaches.

An evident blue vein on the forehead signals enormous stress and problems with the lower burner, which refers to the part of abdomen below the belly button, where the kidneys, bladder, small intestine, and large intestine reside.

Evident bulging blue veins on the bridge of the nose indicate food retention and indigestion.

An evident blue vein at the corners of the mouth or on the chin indicate ailments in the reproductive system.

Bulging, misshapen veins that are dark purple in color indicate a susceptibility to coronary heart disease.

Face twitching. The twitching of the eyelids, corners of the mouth, and facial muscles is often related to emotional factors, and it is more often seen in women than men. The causes of this condition include stagnation of liver *qi*[1], wind pathogen[2] blocking collaterals, liver wind stirring up internally[3], and wind-phlegm obstructing collaterals[4].

Spasms accompanied by lightheadedness and tinnitus indicate a stagnation of liver *qi*.

Sudden spasms accompanied by headaches and tearing up indicate an attack of exogenic wind and cold obstructing the Yangming collateral.

Face twitching and muscle numbing on the affected side are a result of *qi* deficiency due to prolonged illness and wind-phlegm obstructing collateral.

Spider angiomas (spider moles) on the face. A spider mole is one with a small artery at the center surrounded by slender dilated capillaries branching out like spider legs, giving it its name. They

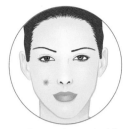

Spider angiomas (spider moles) on the face.

are often found in acute, chronic hepatitis or cirrhosis cases, and pathogenic spider moles can also be seen in pregnant women and healthy people.

Spider moles in women during puberty and pregnancy are a normal condition caused by excessive secretion of female hormones.

The sudden appearances of spider moles in men or elderly women are a probable sign of chronic hepatitis or cirrhosis.

A rapid increase in the number of spider moles signals the worsening of a liver disease.

---

1 Stagnation of liver *qi*. Failure of *qi* movement due to the failure of the liver's dredging and draining functions. Manifestations are primarily depression or short temper, pain, and distension in the lower abdomen.

2 Wind pathogen. Wind pathogens cause illnesses. It occurs year round, but most commonly in spring.

3 Liver wind stirring up internally. Generally referring to ailments caused by wind pathogens, fire/heat, and deficiency of *yin* and blood. The symptoms are mainly twitching limbs, vertigo and tremor.

4 Wind-phlegm obstructing collateral. Wind-phlegm stasis obstructs the meridians and collaterals, characterized by common symptoms such as hemiplegia, facial paralysis, slurred speech or silence, waning or loss of sensation, dizziness and vertigo, heavy and sticky phlegm, and tongue deviations. Often seen in the recovery period after a stroke.

Tips for Caring for Your Face

Eliminating facial puffiness can be done through invigorating the spleen, replenishing the lungs, and improving *qi* circulation to eliminate swelling and clearing away water. Here are some methods:

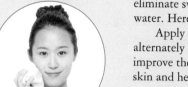

Apply cold and hot towels alternately on your face.

Apply cold and hot towels alternately on your face, which will improve the blood circulation on the skin and help eliminate unwanted water retention in your face.

Eat more foods with properties that promote the flow of water to eliminate swelling, e.g. red beans, coix seeds, and winter melon, which increase metabolism and reduce swelling.

Consume a light diet, eat less foods that are oily or strong in taste, and eat more foods that are low in salt, sugar, and oil.

Maintain a regular schedule of work and rest to ensure that you have enough sleep. Good rest is conducive to regulating the body's metabolism.

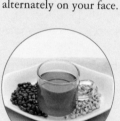

Red beans and coix seeds.

2. Diagnosis Through the Eyes

According to the *Inner Canon of the Yellow Emperor*, the essence of the five *zang* and six *fu* organs all ascend to the eyes, which can reveal the health status of the *zang-fu* organs. This is indicative of the close relationship of the eyes with the *zang-fu* organs, muscle and bone meridians, spirit, and *qi* and blood. The reason the eyes can see everything and differentiate colors is that they are nourished by the essence of the *zang* and *fu* organs. The disharmony of *zang-fu* organs and meridians and collaterals are often reflected in the eyes, even leading to some eye diseases. Conversely, eye diseases can also affect the connected internal organs through meridians and collaterals, even causing a general malaise throughout the body. By observing the eyes, we can not only diagnose eye diseases, but also changes in the internal organs, thereby arriving at diagnoses of other diseases.

Given the close relationship of the eyes with the five *zang* organs and based on the relationship between the eyes and the meridians, the eyes are divided into different parts with regards to the related meridians to show how a particular part of the eye reflects a certain internal organ.

Looking straight ahead, draw an imaginary straight line connecting the centers of the pupils, and then extend it through the medial and lateral canthi, then draw another straight line vertically through the centers of the pupils and extend it beyond the upper and lower eye sockets. In this way, the eye is divided into four parts. Then divide each part further into two equal

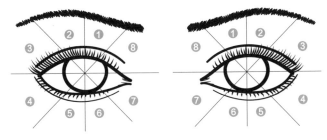

❶ Lungs and large intestine
❷ Kidneys and bladder
❸ Upper burner (including everything above the diaphragm—the thorax, back, the internal organs in chest cavity, neck, head and face, five sense organs, and upper limbs)
❹ Liver and gallbladder
❺ Middle burner (including everything below the diaphragm and above the belly button, the upper abdomen, lower back and back, and all the internal organs)
❻ Heart and small intestine
❼ Spleen and stomach
❽ Lower burner (below the level of the belly button, the lower abdomen, sacrum, illum, hips, pelvis, reproductive and urinary systems, and the lower limbs)

Distribution of corresponding *zang* and *fu* organs in the eyes.

zones, i.e. four quarters and eight identical areas. These eight identical areas are the eight zones, each corresponding to a specific internal organ (refer to the picture on page 31).

The Color of the Eyes

Changes in the color of the eyes are reflective of a person's state of health. By inspecting the color of both eyes and blood streaks in the eyes, a doctor can determine whether there are pathogenic developments with the connected organs. The parts of the eye that are easier to observe include the white of the eye and the iris (or, the black). A clean, bluish white is considered the normal color of the white. If abnormalities occur in the white, e.g. the color turns red, yellow, or has some color spots, this signals problems with your health. If there is a black spot on the iris, you should pay attention to it.

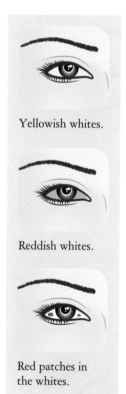

Yellowish whites.

Reddish whites.

Red patches in the whites.

Yellowish whites. If the eyes and your body all look yellowish, it means there is damp-heat in your body. If the body appears yellow, accompanied by low spirits and fatigue, you are most likely experiencing a deficiency of both spleen and blood.

Reddish whites. If the whites look red, accompanied by severe chills and feverish sensations, it means there is heat in the body. If the eyes look red and burn, it indicates that you may be infected with a virus.

Red patches in the whites. Blood patches in the whites are a sign of cerebral arteriosclerosis. If there are small red dots in the whites, you should watch out for the possible onset of diabetes.

Black dots on the iris. When black dots of various sizes appear in the heart zone of the eyes, it suggests the risk of coronary heart disease, myocardial infarction, or heart disease.

Redness in the whites with a tinge of black. This is most often seen in conditions such as a long-time disease that has been treated but never cured, indicating that the pathogen has gone deep in the body and been transformed into a heat causing blood stagnation and blood stasis inside the body. The ailment tends to last a long time and is accompanied by severe blood stasis.

Physical Changes in the Eyes

In addition to diagnosis through observing the color of the eyes, the changes in the physical forms can also be used as criteria for diagnosis. If other abnormalities occur in the eyes, you should address them.

Observing the form of the eyes aims to determine whether the overall physical form of the eyes is normal. If abnormality appears, e.g. abnormally tearing up, puffiness of the eyelids, or abnormalities in the pupils, it may suggest that there is a problem with your health.

Abnormally watery eyes. This is a manifestation of insufficient liver blood. A deficient cold of liver meridian and deficiency of both liver and kidneys may all result in watery eyes.

Abnormalities with the pupils. If one pupil is smaller than the other or one pupil retracts at a slower rate or at a smaller scale, the person may be suffering

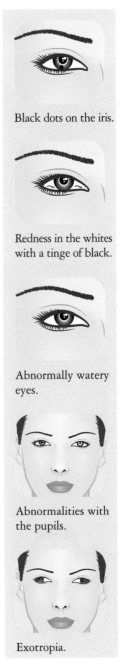

Black dots on the iris.

Redness in the whites with a tinge of black.

Abnormally watery eyes.

Abnormalities with the pupils.

Exotropia.

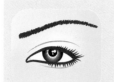

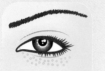

Puffiness of the eyelids.

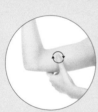

Fat granules.

from cerebral apoplexy.

Exotropia. If both eyes are exotropic, it may indicate cancer or carbon monoxide poisoning. If only one eye is exotropia, it might signal diabetes.

Puffiness of the eyelids. Abnormal metabolism of the kidney and gastrointestine may lead to water retention in the body, leading to puffiness of the eyelids.

Fat granules. Fat granules on the eyelids or around the eyes may indicate that your cholesterol level is too high.

Tips for Caring for Your Eyes

Maintain good eye hygiene. Avoid glaring light that irritates the eyes and do not look at electronic devices such as your mobile phone or TV for a prolonged period. Consume a light diet, and avoid foods with a pungent taste. Maintain a regular schedule of work and rest, and try not to stay up late.

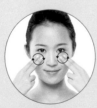

Qingling point.

Massage the Qingling point. The Qingling point[1] regulates *qi*, alleviates pain, soothes the chest, and calms the heart. Pat or press-knead this point often, and it can relieve yellowing of the eyes. It also helps improve the symptoms of neuropathic headaches and angina.

Massage the Chengqi point. The Chengqi point helps those who have uncontrollable watery eyes to improve this symptom. It can also treat eye diseases such as short-sightedness, night blindness, glaucoma, and conjunctivitis.

Chengqi points.

Eliminate fat granules. Keep the eye area clean to ensure the skin's normal function of excretion and absorption. Be careful to consume more light foods and a lower fat diet. Massage the skin surrounding the eyes every day to promote blood circulation and assist the metabolic function of the skin around the eyes.

3. Diagnosis Through the Ears

Although they are a tiny part of the human body, the ears epitomize the various organs and tissues of the body. All human organs and parts have representation points in the ear, revealing the physiological and pathological conditions of the internal organs throughout the body.

TCM holds that the ears are governed by the kidneys, and the kidneys open into the ears. At the same time, the ears are also orifices of the heart, lungs, spleen, and liver. There are abundant vascular nerves beneath the surface of the ears that are inextricably linked with the brain and various parts of the human body.

The distribution of related internal organs in the ears follows some rules. In fact they are arranged on the anterolateral section of the ears like an upside down fetus in the womb, with the head facing down, the arms and lower limbs facing up, and the chest and torso in the middle.

The Color of the Ears

Color changes in the ears may suggest certain illnesses. Keep an eye on the color of your ears and attend to any evident color changes.

Use the thumb and index finger to pull the auricle against the light. Look straight at the auricle and observe the ear from top to bottom, then front to back. Examine it carefully, and

---

1 Acupoint. Acupoints are the specially chosen locations through which *qi* and blood of the *zang* and *fu* organs and the meridians and collaterals are transfused and transported to the body surface. Mainly distributed along the pathways of the meridians and collaterals at points where nerve endings concentrate or thicker nerve fibers pass, they are closely related to the organs and tissues deep inside the human body. Acupoints are the reaction points of the disease and stimulation points for treatment. By stimulating a specific acupoint, the resistance mechanism in the body can be mobilized for the purpose of disease prevention and disease treatment.

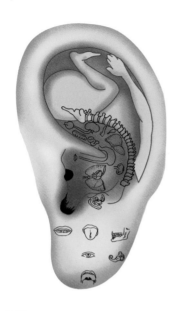

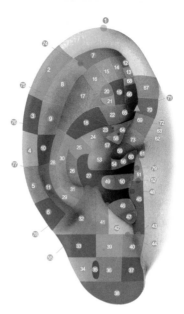

❶ Ear apex
❷ Liver *yang*
❸ Helix 1
❹ Helix 2
❺ Helix 3
❻ Helix 4
❼ Finger
❽ Wrist
❾ Elbow
❿ Shoulder
⓫ Collarbone
⓬ Toe
⓭ Heel
⓮ Ankle
⓯ Knee
⓰ Hip
⓱ Lumbosacral spine
⓲ Abdomen
⓳ Middle triangular fossa
⓴ Shenmen
㉑ Pelvic
㉒ Hip

㉓ Kidney
㉔ Pancreas
㉕ Liver
㉖ Spleen
㉗ Lung
㉘ Thoracic spine
㉙ Cervical spine
㉚ Chest
㉛ Neck
㉜ Occipital bone
㉝ Jaw
㉞ Inner ear
㉟ Cheek
㊱ Eye
㊲ Anterior earlobe
㊳ Tonsil
㊴ Tongue
㊵ Tooth
㊶ Temples
㊷ Forehead
㊸ Anterior intertragic notch
㊹ Posterior intertragic notch

㊺ Lower tragus
㊻ *Sanjiao* (triple burners/energizers)
㊼ Endocrine
㊽ Adrenalin
㊾ Heart
㊿ Trachea
(51) Upper tragus
(52) External nose
(53) Stomach
(54) Cardia
(55) Tragus apex
(56) Esophagus
(57) Duodenum
(58) Small intestine
(59) Ear center
(60) Mouth
(61) External ear
(62) Appendix
(63) Bladder
(64) Large intestine
(65) Sciatic nerve
(66) Internal genitalia
(67) Anus
(68) Superior triangular fossa
(69) Urethra
(70) External genitalia
(71) Sympathetic nerve
(72) Angle of superior concha
(73) Rectum
(74) Fengxi point
(75) Ureter
(76) Center of superior concha
(77) Brainstem
(78) Central rim
(79) Apex of antitragus

Distribution of the *zang* and *fu* organs in the ear.

when spotting a color change, compare it with the other ear to determine the condition.

In general, white is the color of deficiency and cold, yellow is the color of dampness and spleen disease, red mainly indicates heat syndrome, blue signals liver disease, and black mostly points to kidney disease, fluid retention syndrome, and blood stasis. Regardless of what color the ears may look, bright and moist is always a good sign, while dull and shriveling is bad. Once a disease develops, the ear color changes as a result. A bright color suggests a new ailment, while a dull color means the ailment has lasted for some time.

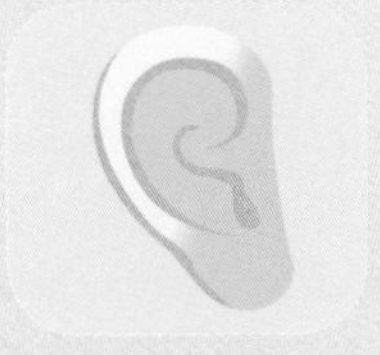

Pale auricle.

Pale auricle. When the auricle looks pale, it indicates deficiency of both *qi* and blood. Rub the ear lobes with your hands, and if they still look pale, it is a sign of anemia.

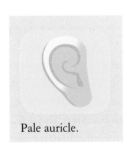

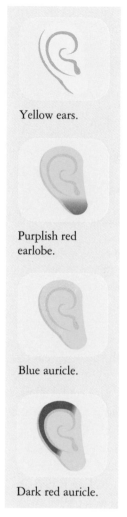

Yellow ears.

Purplish red
earlobe.

Blue auricle.

Dark red auricle.

Yellow ears. When the ear looks yellow and the eyes and face also show a yellow tinge, combined with yellow urine, it usually indicates jaundice.

Purplish red earlobe. When the earlobe appears purplish red, accompanied by swelling and even ulcers that turn into scabs easily, this is the result of high blood sugar in the body.

Blue auricle. If the auricle appears pure blue, it indicates pain and inflammation in the joints. If the auricle looks so blue that it is almost black, this signals a deficiency of kidney qi and blood stasis due to a lengthy illness.

Dark red auricle. If the auricle looks dark red and is accompanied by pain and swelling redness, it indicates hyperactive heat of the liver and gallbladder or fire toxins blazing upward, which is often seen in such illnesses as eczema or otitis media.

Physical Changes in the Ears

Another key aspect of diagnostic ear reading is to observe the changes in the physical shape of the ears. Whether there are nodules or protrusions, and whether there is a foreign body in the ear, all of which are criteria for diagnosing an ailment.

A normal, healthy ear should have stiff ear bones, and the helix should appear smooth and level, while the auricle is meaty and moist without any nodules.

If the ears have bumps or cord-like bumps, spots of depression and a dull appearance, it usually indicates chronic organic diseases such as cirrhosis of the liver and tumors. If

there is pus or bleeding in the ear, this is
a manifestation of a hyperactive liver and
gallbladder heat flaring up, and more
attention is required.

Swelling and aching auricle. A red,
swelling auricle indicates hyperactivity
of wind-heat and liver *yang*, which often
result in symptoms such as coughing, a
stuffy nose, and headaches.

Ear with nodules. If nodules or cord-
like bumps and depressed spots appear in
some part of the ear, it may be a sign of
cirrhosis of the liver and tumors.

Ear bleeding. A sudden burst of blood
that is substantial in volume accompanied
by ear pain means the liver fire is blazing
upward adversely. When the bleeding is
gradual and not substantial in volume, it
suggests hyperactivity of fire due to *yin*
deficiency[1].

Fleshy growth inside the ear.
A tiny fleshy growth in the external
acoustic meatus that is cherry-shaped
with a big head but small stem, also
known as hemorrhoid of the ear, is
mostly caused by heat toxin in the liver
and gallbladder.

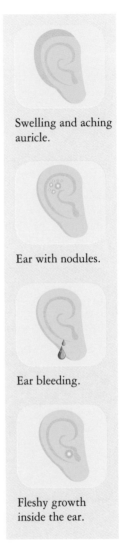

Swelling and aching
auricle.

Ear with nodules.

Ear bleeding.

Fleshy growth
inside the ear.

---

1 Hyperactivity of fire due to *yin* deficiency. Failure of *yin* fluid to
meet the basic needs of a human body leads to the body's declining
capacity to restrict *yang* heat, and as a result a pathogenic condition
occurs in terms of *yang* heat needed for maintaining normal human
activity. This is most closely related to deficiency of liver and kidney
yin due to over-exhaustion, old age, and long-term illness, and
overactive sexual activity.

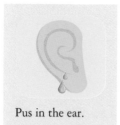

Pus in the ear.

Pus in the ear. When there is pus in the ear, it is usually the result of wind-heat disturbing upward[1], damp-heat of the liver and gallbladder, or deficiency of the kidney *yin*[2] leading to the flaring up of deficient fire[3].

Tips for Caring for Your Ears

Pull the earlobe downward. Frequently massaging the ear helps dredge the meridians and channels to enhance the flow of *qi* and blood, strengthening the kidneys and lower back. You can do this by pulling upward on the apex of the auricle and pulling downward on the earlobe, then pressing the tragus.

Press-knead the Taichong point. An acupoint that soothes the liver, regulates blood, and clears the meridians. The Taichong point is effective for preventing ear bleeding. Frequent massaging of this point helps relieve dizziness, insomnia, and high blood pressure.

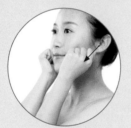

Pull the earlobe downward.

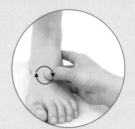

Taichong point.

---

4. Diagnosis Through the Nose

As the entrance to the respiratory passage, the nose connects the inside of the human body directly with the outside world. Many acupoints are located on the surface of the nose. At the onset of an illness, the color and the physical form of the nose will change accordingly. Those tiny changes can help people diagnose for themselves what ailments are developing.

Diagnostic nose reading refers to the method of observing the color and luster of the nose, its physical form, and behavioral changes in the course of breathing to determine the underlying ailment. It is an important component of TCM diagnosis.

The nose is the orifice of the lungs and the entrance to the perspiration passage. The five internal organs all ascent their *qi* to the nose—a prime example of all visceral organs and tissues in the body. Each *zang* and *fu* organ and tissue shares a corresponding site on the nose. For example, the tip of the nose reflects the health of the spleen. If the tip of the nose is red or shows some abnormalities, it may indicate problems with the spleen. As shown in the picture on the top of page 42, the different parts of the nose correspond to the related *zang-fu* organs on the nose. They reflect, systematically and selectively, the physiological and pathological conditions of the viscera.

---

1 Wind-heat disturbing upward. Wind-heat pathogen flares upward to disturb orifices such as the head and eyes, manifesting symptoms such as hot sensations, chills, headache, lightheadedness, and coughing.
2 Kidney *yin*. In contrast to kidney *yang*, kidney *yin* pacifies, moisturizes, nourishes, and forms shapes. It can also restrain the hyperactivity of *yang*.
3 Deficient fire. A pathological phenomenon of overconsumption of *yin* leading to an exuberance of fire. Deficient fire is the pathogenesis of syndrome of hyperactivity of fire due to *yin* deficiency. The causes of the syndrome include congenital insufficiency, long-term illness, over-exertion, over-active sexual activity, anxiety and worry, and the exogenous heat damaging *yin* fluid. The manifestations are mainly hot sensations in the body, feverish sensations in the chest, palms, and soles, night sweats, emaciation, dry mouth and throat, and restlessness. Flaring up of deficient fire. Deficiency of kidney *yin* leads to a failure of water to restrain fire, which results in hyperactivity of fire. Symptoms include sore throat, lightheadedness and vertigo, irritability and insomnia, tinnitus and forgetfulness, warm sensations in the palms and soles, or redness in the eyes, and ulcers in the mouth and on the tongue.

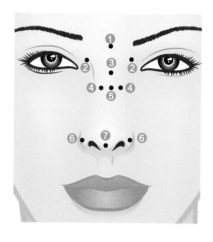

① Lung
② Breast
③ Heart
④ Gallbladder
⑤ Liver
⑥ Stomach
⑦ Spleen

The distribution of the corresponding *zang-fu* organs.

The Color of the Nose

The nose is one of the more complete and visible parts that is representative of the holographic phenomenon of the human body. By observing the color changes of different parts of the nose, pathogenic changes can be detected in the viscera that corresponds to that part of the nose.

The nose of a healthy person is bright and pinkish, similar to that of the ears, although with slight differences in shade. In

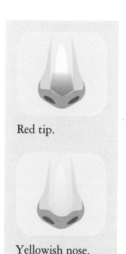

Red tip.

Yellowish nose.

addition, it is shiny and without pimples or bumps. If an ailment develops in the body, the color of the nose will change. The darker the nose, the more serious the ailment.

Red tip. When the tip of the nose is red, it suggests excessive heat[1] of the spleen and lungs. When it is slightly red, it means there is deficient heat[2] of the spleen meridian. When the edge of the nostril is red, it indicates ailments in the intestines.

Yellowish nose. When the nose looks yellow, it means there is damp-heat in the body. If it is combined with a yellow color in the face and eyes, it is symptomatic of jaundice, and is often seen in acute jaundice hepatitis.

Pale nose. This is often a sign of deficiency of *qi* and blood. If the tip of the nose is pale with white millet-like bumps, this often indicates irregular menstruation.

Bluish black tip. This is a sign of pain, often abdominal pain. Women with a great volume of dark red menstrual blood often experience painful menstrual periods.

Bluish nose. Scholars have found that people are likely to have the onset of ailments with the spleen and pancreas when their noses look bluish, brown, or black.

Physical Changes in the Nose

Changes in the physical shape of the nose are also indicative of the pathological changes in the viscera, which can often be determined by observing the outward appearance of the nose, whether there are spots on the nose, and whether there is anything unusual in the secretion of mucus.

The nose of a normal, healthy person is usually proportionate

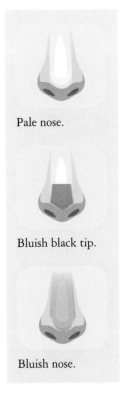

Pale nose.

Bluish black tip.

Bluish nose.

---

1 Excessive heat. Invasion of heat pathogen into the human body from the exterior to the interior. Clinical symptoms are high fever and preference of cold, thirst and preference of cold drink, redness in the face and eyes, irritability or delirium, abdominal fullness and aversion to pressure, constipation, scanty dark urine, red tongue and yellow, dry coating.

2 Deficient heat. Often caused by internal injury due to degeneration, such as depletion of essence and *qi* due to long-time illness, and overexertion, which lead to the imbalance and weakening of *zang-fu* organs and bring about internal heat that evolves into deficient fire.

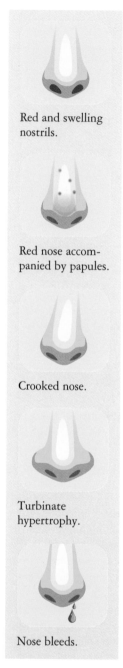

Red and swelling nostrils.

Red nose accompanied by papules.

Crooked nose.

Turbinate hypertrophy.

Nose bleeds.

in size, with a straight ridge and a good outward appearance, all of which indicate good health. Abnormalities occurring with the physical form of the nose usually mean that there are problems with the person's health. The changes in the behavior of the nose also reflect some internal diseases in the human body, e.g. a frequent runny nose may suggest chronic rhinitis, which deserves attention.

Red and swelling nostrils. This is often caused by endogenous heat, mainly found in the initial onset of nasal sores, boils, furuncles, or eczema.

Red nose accompanied by papules. The tip of the nose may be red, accompanied by papules, and the affected skin may become thicker after a while and turns purplish red. This is often caused by stomach heat fuming upwards to the lungs and blood clogging the lung meridian.

Crooked nose. A crooked nose is often associated with the foot, and is often accompanied by foot pain. It is also seen in people with facial paralysis.

Turbinate hypertrophy. The hypertrophy of the inferior and middle turbinates is often caused by mucosal hyperaemia or blood stasis. It is likely a symptom of the onset of diabetes or gout.

Nose bleeds. Nose bleeds may be caused by wind-heat clogging of the lung, hyperactivity of stomach fire, liver fire flaring up and affecting the lung, or a deficiency of kidney *yin*[1].

Tips for Caring for Your Nose

Wash your nasal cavity with cold water to improve the blood circulation in the nose and prevent the onset of common colds and respiratory ailments. You can also massage the nose. Use your thumb and index finger to pinch the base of the nose and push and pull it up and down 12 times, which will enhance the resistance of the nasal mucosa.

Alleviate redness in the nose. Your nose becomes red because there is some problem with your spleen and stomach, such as excessive heat in the spleen and stomach. Massaging the Zusanli and Neiting points can relieve heat in the stomach. Massage for five minutes twice or three times a day.

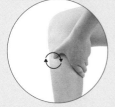

Zusanli point.

Nosebleed. When your nose bleeds, assume a reclining position, and the blood will collect and congeal at the front part of the nasal cavity, which is conducive to stopping the bleeding. Do not tilt your head backward, which will cause the blood to reverse back to the mouth or throat and flow into the stomach, leading to symptoms such as nausea and vomiting. Alternatively, you can massage the Yingxiang point, which helps clear the orifice and invigorate the meridians and stop the bleeding. Massaging this point can also relieve nosebleeds and symptoms such as a stuffy nose, rhinitis, and facial paralysis.

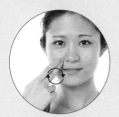

Yingxiang point.

---

1 Deficiency of kidney *yin*. A deficiency of kidney *yin* leads to its failure to restrain *yang*, and as a result deficient heat and fire disturb throughout the interior of the body, or disturb the blood and mind, as well as developing pathological changes in the brain, bones, teeth, and head hair, and a failure to nourish the organs and orifices. It is mostly caused by long-term illness, overactive sexual activity, long-term lack of sleep and unhealthy dietary habits. Symptoms are a feverish sensation in the chest, palms, and soles, tidal fever, night sweat, soreness and aching in the lower back and knees, dizziness and vertigo, tinnitus, insomnia and dreaminess, nocturnal emissions, reduced amount of menstrual blood, or amenorrhea.

5. Diagnosis Through the Lips

The lips are closely related to the health of a human being. Observing the color and physical changes of the lips can help determine the physiological and pathological changes of the viscera and thereby the possible onset of certain illnesses.

TCM holds that the lips have a very close relation with organs such as the spleen, stomach, large intestine, and liver. The lips can thus reflect the state of the essence of the viscera. Modern medical science also believes that the lips, which are rich in blood capillaries, can quickly reveal ailments in the viscera.

The lips are a hub of fourteen meridians and a center of communication for the viscera. The picture below shows how the corresponding *zang-fu* organs are distributed on the lips.

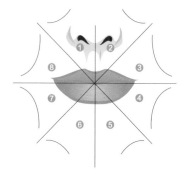

❶ Small intestine and heart
❷ Middle burner
❸ Liver and gallbladder
❹ Upper burner
❺ Kidney and bladder
❻ Lung and large intestine
❼ Lower burner
❽ Spleen and stomach

The distribution of the corresponding *zang-fu* organs on the lips.

The Color of the Lips

Examining the color of the lips is the method by which physiological and pathological changes of the human internal organs can be observed through the colors and gloss of the lips, which allows for early diagnosis of the diseases that are developing in the human body.

The normal healthy color of the lips is light pink, but it may change slightly due to differences in a person's constitution and age. When people are sick, the color of their lips varies based on the types of diseases they are suffering from. For example, patients with heart disease tend to have dark purple lips.

Pale lips. Pale lips are more often found in patients with anemia. If the lips are pale and dry, you should beware of the possibility of diabetes.

Red lips. Bright red lips means damp-heat in the *zang* and *fu* organs. A dark red lower lip indicates deficiency of the spleen. If the lips are dark purple with a tinge of red, it is a sign of stagnation of *qi* and blood stasis[1].

Yellowish lips. This is often associated with an unrestrained and unsanitized diet and picky eating habits, combined with dampness heat lodged in the liver and spleen. The symptoms include low spirits and weariness, tired extremities, and dizziness.

Black lips. When the lips are grayish black, it suggests a stomach *yang* deficiency in the middle burner. When the lips are slightly black with a tinge of purplish red, it indicates stasis in the body. When the lips are purplish black, it means there is a blood stasis flowing toward the heart.

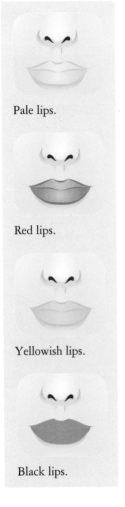

Pale lips.

Red lips.

Yellowish lips.

Black lips.

---

1 Stagnation of *qi* and blood stasis. A pathological state in which both *qi* stagnation and blood stasis are present. In general, the initial imbalance of *qi* flow leads to problems with blood circulation, causing blood stasis and stagnation to occur. The condition can be a result of emotional stress, improper diet, or long-term illness in the elderly and is manifested as chest and flank fullness and compression, mobile pain or stabbing pain, localized pain averse to touch, and pain that is sensitive to touch, or hard lumps, with some localized parts swelling and turning bluish purple.

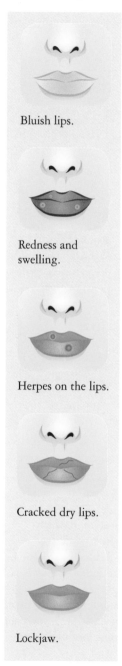

Bluish lips.

Redness and swelling.

Herpes on the lips.

Cracked dry lips.

Lockjaw.

Bluish lips. Bluish lips signify stagnation of *qi* and blood stasis, signaling that the person is susceptible to acute onset such as vascular embolism.

The Physical Changes in the Lips

The lips are closely related to the spleen, which is the root of the acquired constitution. The health of the human body can thus be judged by observing the lips. The physical state of the lips is inseparable from that of the mouth. The physical state of the lips are judged by their shapes, whether they are dry or moist, or whether there are bumps or sores on the lips, along with other factors. For example, dry lips are caused by fluid depletion due to dryness-heat, and ulcers on the lips are often the result of hyperactive fire or a viral infection. Behavioral changes in the mouth, such as a crooked mouth and lips, are also symptoms of abnormality.

Redness and swelling. The lips are red and swelling, with a sore on the highest part of the swelling, and the sore is hard and painful, which results from the clogging of evil toxins.

Herpes on the lips. Small ulcers growing on the lips, with a yellow fluid and scabs that develop in a few days are a sign of the onset of cold, pneumonia, or measles.

Cracked dry lips. The lips are dry and cracked, with small flakes on the surface or even deep cracks. This is the result of fluid depletion due to dryness-heat.

Lockjaw. Diseases such as epilepsy and tetanus, and acute infantile convulsions could all be the cause for lockjaw.

Drooping mouth. Drooping mouth, with the tongue deviating to one side and often accompanied by drooling, is likely a sign of facial paralysis or cerebral stroke.

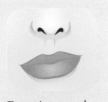

Drooping mouth.

Tips for Caring for Your Lips

Pale lips. This often result from insufficient blood and *qi* leading to failure of the blood to nourish the lips. Consume a diet rich in iron, e.g. eat foods such as animal livers and spinach more often to replenish the blood. In addition, exercise on a regular basis to be physically strong and promote the circulation of *qi* and blood. Pale lips are often seen in people suffering from anemia. The Sanyinjiao point can be massaged frequently to replenish the spleen and augment blood, regulate the liver and tone the kidney, replenish *qi*, and nourish blood. Frequent massaging of the Sanyinjiao point will help relieve anemia caused by insufficient blood and *qi*. It also works quite well for women suffering from anemia due to such conditions as metrorrhagia and postpartum hemorrhages.

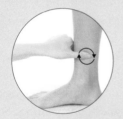

Sanyinjiao point.

Dry, scaly lips. Drink more water to replenish body fluids in a timely way. Apply lip balms to keep the lips moist and prevent them from flaking. Consume a diet rich in fresh vegetables, fruits, and supplementary vitamins. Do not lick your lips, because that will make them even drier. In addition, massaging the Zusanli point can help invigorate the middle burner and augment *qi* and clear the meridians and collaterals to promote the circulation of *qi* and blood. Use the pads of both thumbs to press the Zusanli point alternately until a distension is produced. Do it 30 to 50 times a day until a localized distension is felt. Long-term massaging of this acupoint can help keep your lips red.

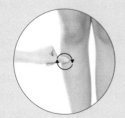

Zusanli point.

6. Diagnosis Through the Tongue

Tongue diagnosis is one of the ways to detect diseases in traditional Chinese medicine, and the tongue coating is particularly important in this method. From the perspective of TCM theory, the color of the tongue reveals the nature of the disease and the status of the vital *qi*. The tongue coating can also tell the depth the pathogenic *qi* has penetrated into the body and detect the presence or absence of stomach *qi*. The moistness of the tongue coating indicates changes in the six climatic exopathogens and the possible damage that has been done to body fluids.

TCM teaches that the tongue is an orifice where early signs of problems manifest and to which many meridians and collaterals in the human body are connected. Therefore, the body's meridians and *zang-fu* organ, the 4-levels theory of *ying* (nutrient)-*wei* (defense)-*qi* (vital energy)-*xue* (blood), the external and internal, the *yin* and *yang*, cold and heat, and deficiency and excess, all are reflected in the tongue. Being the result of fumigation by the stomach *qi*, the tongue coating manifests the changes in the tongue mucosa. All five *zang* organs receive *qi* from the stomach, so the tongue can be used as a means to determine the health status of the five *zang* organs, detecting cold or heat and deficiency or excess. Tongue diagnosis relies mainly on the changes that happen to the tongue's shape, color, dryness, and coating. Such information will uncover the nature of the pathogen, help differentiate the types of syndromes of *ying-wei-qi-xue*, and determine the extent of the body fluid.

The tongue consists of four parts, the tip, center, root, and sides. TCM further divides the tongue body into the upper, middle, and lower burners, with the tip serving as the upper burner, the middle as the middle burner, and the root as the lower burner. The relation between the tongues's parts and the *zang* and *fu* organs is that the tip connects to the heart and lungs, the middle connects to the spleen and stomach, the sides of the tongue connect to the liver and gallbladder, and the root

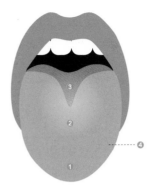

❶ Tip: upper burner, heart and lungs
❷ Middle: middle burner, spleen and stomach
❸ Root: lower burner, kidneys
❹ Sides: liver and gallbladder

The distribution of pertaining *zang* and *fu* organs in the tongue.

connects to the kidneys. See the illustration above.

When conducting a tongue diagnosis, attention should be paid to some confounding external factors to avoid misdiagnosis. Instead of using a dim electrical light at night, soft natural light during the day is recommended. Maintain a sitting position during the tongue examination. Stick out the tongue naturally, keep it relaxed, level out the tongue surface, and let the tongue body droop naturally. Certain foods and drugs can affect the color of the tongue coating, presenting a false color. You should ask more questions in order to truthfully identify its color. The condition of the oral cavity may also affect the appearance of the tongue. For example, missing teeth can result in a thicker tongue coating on the affected side, crowns can leave teeth impression on the sides of the tongue, and those who breathe through the mouth while sleeping may develop a thicker tongue coating. To avoid misdiagnosis, you should exercise caution while examining the tongue.

The Shape and Surface of the Tongue

Different shapes of the tongue and the presence of red spots on the tongue are factors associated with the health status of the *zang-fu* organs. Therefore, observing the shape and surface of the tongue is an important aspect of diagnostic tongue reading.

Red spots on the tongue. Red spots on the tongue surface become noticeable because of the swelling of the tongue papilla

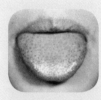

Red spots on the tongue.

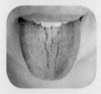

Cracks on the tongue surface.

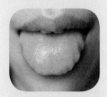

Teeth impressions on the tongue.

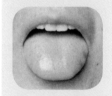

Bulky tongue body.

caused by inflammation. They are not raised above the tongue surface under normal circumstances. If the tongue papilla are enlarged and become prickled, it indicates hyperactive endogenous heat in the body, signaling that there may be inflammation in the body.

Red spots and prickles on tip of tongue indicate exuberance of heart fire[1].

Red spots and prickles on center of tongue indicate hyperactive gastrointestinal fire.

Red spots and prickles on sides of tongue indicate exuberance of heat disturbing the liver and gallbladder internally.

Red spots with depression, little and very dry tongue coating signal the deterioration of a chronic disease.

Cracks on the tongue surface. Cracks like gullies appear on the tongue surface. They may be horizontal, vertical, or shaped like the Chinese character)||, with no coating in the cracks. Such sign on the tongue mostly results from endogenous heat in the body depleting the body of fluid, and essence and blood are so deficient that they cannot nourish the tongue.

Horizontal cracks indicate *yin* deficiency due to old age.

Dark red tongue without coating or with horizontal cracks is indicative of *yin* deficiency and depletion of body fluid.

Cracks shaped like)|| indicate excessive heat in the body.

Pale light tongue with cracks indicate deficiency of essence and blood.

Dark red tongue with fissures on sides and tip indicate

flaring up of heart fire[2].

Teeth impressions on the tongue. The tongue body is bulkier than usual. When sticking out, it fills the whole mouth and its edge is uneven due to teeth impressions. If the body of the tongue appears pale, along with the coating, it indicates a deficiency of kidney *yang*, and there is water dampness, phlegm, and fluid retention.

Pale, moist tongue with teeth impressions indicate exuberance and stagnation of cold-dampness.

Pale red tongue with teeth impressions indicate spleen deficiency.

Red, swelling tongue with teeth impressions on the sides indicate turbid phlegm[3] stagnation.

Glossy tongue surface, enlarged, round and tender tongue body, with teeth impressions on the sides indicate spleen *yang* deficiency.

Bulky tongue body. When the body of the tongue is clearly thicker and bulkier than usual and the tongue fills the whole mouth when sticking out, it suggests a deficiency and decline of spleen *yang*, or it may be combined with cold-dampness, causing the tongue body to become enlarged, floaty, tender and pale in color. It often has teeth impressions, too. This is a sign

---

1 Exuberance of heart fire. Hyperactive heat disturbs the heart and mind. Common symptoms include a feverish sensation and thirst, irritability and insomnia, or delirium, constipation, yellow urine, redness in the face, red tongue with yellow coating.

2 Flaring up of heart fire. Exuberance of heat in the heart meridian flares up to the mouth and tongue, leading to common symptoms such as a feverish sensation and thirst, irritability, ulcers in the mouth and tongue that may fester and are painful, and redness in the face.

3 Turbid phlegm. Due to the failure of the spleen's function of transportation and transformation, water stagnates and dampness congestion turns into phlegm, obstructing the flow of *qi*. Clinical manifestations are coughing and shortness of breath, profuse phlegm expectoration, nausea and dizziness, or slippery localized lumps.

of a deficiency syndrome, which includes a spleen or kidney deficiency.

Bulky tongue body with teeth impressions on the sides, thin white coating indicate fluid retention syndrome and phlegm-dampness[1] stagnation.

Pale and bulky tongue body with glossy surface indicate deficiency of spleen *yang* and kidney *yang*.

Bulky and tender tongue body with teeth impressions on the sides indicate water diffusion due to kidney deficiency.

Bulky tongue body with yellow greasy coating indicate damp-heat and phlegm and fluid retention[2] rising upward.

The Color of the Tongue

Observing the color of the tongue is also an important criterion of this diagnostic examination. A healthy person's tongue is usually pale red. If the tongue looks red, it means there is heat in the body. If the tongue is pale, it means that there is cold in the body and a deficiency is possible. If the tongue appears purple, it means blood stasis in the body. Different colors of the tongue reflect different health conditions in the human body.

Pale tongue. This refers to a color that is lighter than normal, or more white and less red, or even completely bloodless. This is because insufficient *yang* results in the weakening transformation function of blood *yin* and a weakened flow of blood. As a result, the blood cannot fully nourish the tongue, rendering it pale and white, which is an indication of deficiency of both *qi* and blood.

Pale tongue texture, bulky and tender, with teeth impressions indicates decline of *yang*.

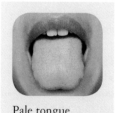
Pale tongue.

Pale tongue texture, slightly shrunken in size indicates deficiency of both *qi* and blood.

Light but still visibly red tongue indicates early phase of deficiency syndrome.

Parched white, bloodless tongue with white lips and gums indicates more severe deficiency syndrome.

Bright red tongue. When the tongue

is bright red, i.e. darker than normal, it is called red tongue, indicating a heat syndrome, which is due to retention of hyperactive heat in the body leading to fluid depletion.

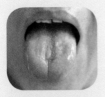

Bright red tongue.

Red tongue tip with prickles indicates flaring up of heart fire.

Red tongue with yellow and dry coating indicates excessive heat in the body.

Red tongue body with little or no coating indicates endogenous heat due to *yin* deficiency.

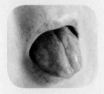

Purplish red tongue.

Red tongue side indicates mostly hyperactivity of heat in the liver and gallbladder.

Purplish red tongue. When the tongue body becomes dark red, it is a sign that heat pathogen has invaded the blood. Due to the hyperactive *yang* and heat, *qi* and blood flow accelerates and fill the meridians and collaterals to the brim, resulting in a bright red or purplish red tongue body. This is often associated with factors such as high fever, dehydration, coma, or vitamin

---

1 Phlegm-dampness. The disorder of the spleen's function in transportation and transformation leads to the disharmony of distribution and circulation of the body fluid, leading to water-dampness stagnation internally, which in turn leads to dampness and turbidity stagnating in the body, generating phlegm over time, with phlegm and turbidity obstructing the lung's function. Major symptoms are coughing with profuse phlegm expectoration, white sputum, and tightness of the chest.

2 Phlegm and fluid retention. Failure to be properly transported and fully transformed for good use, water stagnates in certain areas, which is the result of an attack of exogenous cold and dampness, improper diet, and overexertion leading to physical deficiency. The symptoms include coughing, wheezing, tightness of chest, and a greasy tongue coating. Sometimes the patient may not cough sputum, but the ailment is manifested as dizziness.

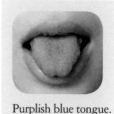

Purplish blue tongue.

deficiency.

Purplish red tongue, dry body, with prickles or cracks indicate hyperactivity of endogenous heat penetrating to the nutritive and blood stages, which is a syndrome of excessive heat.

Dull color with little tongue coating or some cracks indicates syndrome of *yin* deficiency.

Purplish red in tongue center indicates spleen and gastric heat.

Pale tongue with a tinge of red indicates mostly hyperactivity of deficient fire.

Purplish blue tongue. Part or whole tongue body looks purplish blue, which is called purplish blue tongue. This type of tongue signals a dysfunction of the flow of *qi* and blood, resulting in the tongue looking purplish blue. It is often related to venous stasis, slow blood circulation, obstruction of micro-circulation, lack of oxygen, and a deformity of the capillaries.

Whole tongue looking light purplish blue, smooth and moist, shrunken tongue body indicate invasion of cold pathogen leading to a state of *yang* deficiency due to *yin* excess[1].

Whole or sides of tongue looking purplish blue and dull, with blood stasis spots on the sides indicates blood stasis obstructing collaterals.

The tongue often appearing purple indicates a warning sign of the onset of cancer.

Tongue Coating

The different signs observed in the tongue's coating result from stomach *qi*, on which all *zang* and *fu* organs rely. The changes in the tongue coating can thus reflect the health conditions of the viscera, whether syndromes of cold, heat, deficiency, or excess, as well as the nature of the pathogens and the depth of the pathological development in the body.

White coating. This color usually manifests superficies and cold syndromes. White coating is seen in a variety of situations and therefore is not the sole criterion for diagnosis. Other tongue signs, such as the dryness and moistness of the coating, the different shades of color of the tongue texture, and general symptoms, should all be taken into consideration.

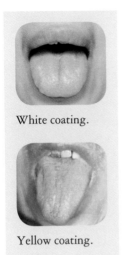

White coating.

Yellow coating.

Thin, white and dry coating indicates heat syndrome or dry pathogen attack.

Thick, white and dry coating indicates dampness turning into heat damaging the fluid.

Pale white coating, glossy and moist indicates cold syndrome or cold-dampness syndrome.

Glossy white coating, sticky and greasy indicates phlegm-dampness stagnated in the spleen.

Glossy, putrid white coating indicates heat accumulation stagnating the stomach.

Yellow coating. There are different shades of yellow tongue coatings, such as light yellow, tender yellow, dark yellow, and light brown. They are often distributed at the tongue's root and center, but can also appear across the whole tongue. A yellow tongue coating is mainly the result of an interior or heat syndrome. Differences should also be noted in the degrees of thickness, dryness, and putridness of yellow tongue coatings.

Thin, light yellow, dry coating indicates excess of interior heat.

---

1 *Yang* deficiency due to *yin* excess. Long-term inception of cold-dampness or ingestion of raw, cold foods results in hyperactivity of *yin* and cold, which depletes *yang*. Clinical symptoms are cold body and limbs, aversion to cold and preference for warmth, weariness, long, and clear urine, loose stool, feeling physically cold, and localized cold pain.

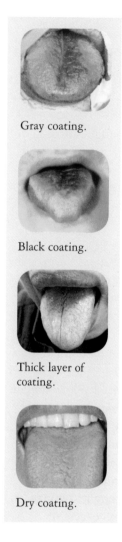

Gray coating.

Black coating.

Thick layer of coating.

Dry coating.

Yellow tongue coating, dry with prickles and cracks indicates depletion of the body fluid and extreme heat in the *zang* and *fu* organs due to extreme hyperactive interior heat.

Thick, yellow and greasy coating indicates food retention or damp-heat accumulated internally.

Yellow, glossy and moist coating indicates manifestation of *yang* deficiency.

Gray coating. Gray tongue coating comes after white or yellow coating, but before black coating arrives, and it is most often seen in patients with chronic or long-term illness or stagnation of liver *qi*, disharmony of the liver and stomach, or disharmony of the spleen and stomach.

Thin, gray, glossy, moist coating indicates cold-dampness congested internally.

Yellowish gray, dry coating indicates febrile illnesses or hyperactivity of fire due to *yin* deficiency.

Whitish gray coating indicates the declining function of the internal organs.

Black coating. When a layer of black coating appears on the tongue surface, it is often the result of the transformation from yellow or gray coating. It indicates that the condition is extremely severe or is likely to become chronic. According to the thickness and degree of moistness on the tongue coating, black coating can be further classified into thin black coating, dry black coating, and thick greasy black coating.

Thin, black coating indicates the condition is quite severe.

Dry black coating indicates fluid depletion due to hyperactive heat.

Dry black coating at the tip of the tongue indicates hyperactivity of heart fire.

Glossy and moist black coating indicates *yang* deficiency leading to extreme hyperactivity of *yin* and cold.

Thick greasy black coating indicates over-active heat pathogen and dampness.

In addition to inspecting the color of the tongue coating for diseases, the thickness, dryness, and presence of coating should also be taken into consideration. The changes in the thickness of tongue coating is indicative of the status of evil *qi* and vital *qi* in the body, as well as the severity of the disease.

Thick layer of coating. Thickness is measured in comparison with your normal coating. When you cannot see the color of the tongue texture through the coating, it means the condition has become more severe or there is gastric retention. Observing the thickness of tongue coating is conducive to determining the prosperity or decline of vital *qi* or evil *qi* and the severity of the condition.

Thick, yellow dry coating indicates depletion of *yin* due to excessive heat.

Thick and greasy white coating indicates cold-dampness obstructions of the spleen and stomach.

Thick, powder-like white coating indicates retention of cold-phlegm[1].

Coating growing thick indicates the condition becomes more severe.

Coating growing thin indicates the condition is improving.

Dry coating. The tongue coating that is dry and lacks fluid, which is called dry coating. In severe cases, dry cracks may appear in the coating. Inflammation or chronic disease tend to have excessive heat accumulated in the body, leading to the

1 Cold-phlegm. Stagnation of cold pathogen and turbid phlegm, characterized by symptoms such as expectorating white sputum, chest tightness and epigastric distension, shortness of breath and wheezing, and chills and cold limbs.

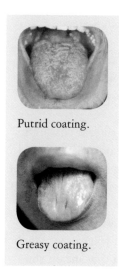

Putrid coating.

Greasy coating.

depletion of fluid. The tongue cannot be nourished by fluid and turns dry as a result.

Dry coating with a white tinge indicates poor water and fluid circulation in the body.

Dry coating, yellow in color indicates hyperactivity of stomach fire.

Dry coating, black in color indicates fluid depletion due to extreme heat.

Dry coating, black in color, with prickles indicates extreme heat exuberance drying up body fluid.

Putrid coating. This refers to a thick coating with big, rough, loose bumps, which is thick at the center and both sides of the tongue, like beancurd residues piling up on the tongue surface that are easy to scrape off. This mostly indicates a heat syndrome, manifested as excess of endogenous heat.

Dull and putrid coating, with white or yellow color is often seen in food retention, turbid phlegm, and a dampness heat syndrome.

Abscess-like coating, i.e. abscess putrid coating indicates deterioration of an internal abscess[1].

Membrane of white coating or erosion, i.e. mouldy, putrid coating is often seen in patients experiencing damp-warm[2], warm-toxin[3], diarrhea, and infantile malnutrition[4].

Greasy coating. This refers to tiny particles closely distributed and evenly forming into patches, attached closely to the tongue surface. It is thick at the center and thin on the sides, and not easily scraped off. This sign indicates stagnation of dampness and turbidity, manifested as phlegm dampness and food retention.

White, smooth, greasy coating indicates mostly phlegm-dampness or deficiency of stomach *yang*.

Thick and greasy yellow coating indicates phlegm-heat[5],

damp-heat, and retention of food.

Thick, greasy coating, not smooth, white as if thickly powdered indicates external evil invasion, accompanied by dampness.

White, greasy coating, not dry, and self-reported sensation of oppression in chest indicates severe dampness due to deficiency of the spleen.

White, thick, slimy coating and sweet taste in the mouth indicates damp-heat of the spleen and stomach.

7. Diagnosis Through the Teeth

Although it is only a tiny part of the human body, the teeth are an important organ. If something goes wrong with the teeth, it does not mean that the teeth alone are diseased. There may also be problems with the viscera. Observing the teeth can help

---

1 Internal abscess. Abscess growing in the *zang* and *fu* organs.

2 Damp-warm. Warm diseases caused by the attack of damp-heat. Initial symptoms are self-claimed feverish sensation, though the skin is not hot to the touch, and fullness and tightness of the epigastrium and abdomen. The pathogen takes time to develop and the illness lasts a long time and lingers on. The center of the pathological development is the spleen and stomach. Warm diseases occur year round, but most often at the end of summer and early fall when it is hot and rains frequently.

3 Warm-toxin. An acute inflammation due to the attack of warm-heat and seasonal toxins. Clinical manifestations are characterized by high fever, swelling and painful head and face or sore throat, and hemorrhagic rashes.

4 Infantile malnutrition (*gan ji* in Chinese). The disease progresses to the mid-phase with complicated conditions of both excess and deficiency and is characterized by evident emaciation, sallow complexion, bloated abdomen and bulging blue veins, and low spirits.

5 Phlegm-heat. Caused by the combination of turbid phlegm and heat evil. Its clinical symptoms are coughing yellow sputum, a feverish sensation, and thirst.

Tips for Caring for Your Tongue

Pale tongue. This is mostly the result of deficiency of *qi* and *yang*. To improve the tongue color, focus on restoring the deficiency and dispelling cold, invigorating *qi* to generate blood. Expose your back more often to the sun for its warmth. People with *yang* deficiency usually experience cold stagnation, so basking in the sun may help them replenish *yang*. It is recommended that people with a deficiency of *qi* and blood and a deficiency of *yang* should drink black tea, which warms the stomach, stimulates the spirit, warms *yang*, and invigorates *qi*. Massaging the Baihui point for 3 to 5 minutes every day will invigorate the *yang* in the governor vessel, thus toning *qi* and restoring the *yang* throughout the body. Gently scraping the skin on the back with Gua Sha therapy can also stimulate the *yang* of the back to replenish the *yang* throughout the body.

Black tongue coating. With black coating, therapies should focus on the aspects of diet, regulating work, a good rest schedule, and TCM treatment to strengthen the body's resistance. In addition, avoid foods with heat properties, such as spicy, pungent, and fried foods. Frequently consume vitamin-rich foods such as fruits and vegetables. Also, drink water with ginseng slices and red dates (Chinese dates or jujube fruits), as ginseng can replenish the original *qi*, while red dates can promote blood circulation and tone the blood. If the black coating is thick and greasy, frequently massage the Neiguan point to help relieve blood stasis and smooth the flow of *qi* and blood. Exercise more, with adequate amounts of time and intensity. It is best to just warm up until you perspire slightly.

Thick white coating. When the coating is thick and white, it indicates cold-dampness stagnation in the spleen and stomach. Therapeutic treatment focuses on warming the middle burner and toning the spleen. Frequently consume foods such as Chinese yams, mushrooms, chestnuts, and red dates, which tone the spleen, strengthen the stomach, nourish the blood, and tranquilize the mind. Eat less raw and cold foods, such as ice cream and ice popsicles, to prevent the cold from attacking the stomach. Do moxibustion at the Guanyuan point for 10 to 15 minutes every day to replenish *yang* and relieve symptoms of cold deficiencies in the spleen and stomach. Brush your teeth every day after you get up in the morning and before going to bed at night. Use salty water or mouthwash to rinse your mouth after each meal to keep your mouth clean.

people get a rough idea of the status of the *zang-fu* organs.

Teeth have a close relationship with the viscera. The "Meridians" chapter in the *Inner Canon of the Yellow Emperor* points out that teeth are not only inseparable from the stomach and large intestine, but are also closely connected to the other internal organs in the human body. The *Inner Canon of the Yellow Emperor* not only affirmed the physiological connection between the teeth and the kidney *qi*, the essence, and the Yangming meridian of the hand and foot, but it also spotted the pathological relationship between the teeth and the viscera, e.g. a toothache is caused by stomach fire, and the loosening or loss of teeth is due to a kidney deficiency. It is not hard, therefore, to see how a single tooth can reflect the health of the body's internal organs.

Based on TCM and modern anatomy, the teeth are classified into incisors, canines, premolars, and molars. The differences in shape and function of the teeth dictate the different internal organs pertaining to the teeth in different locations. The upper incisor connects to the heart, the lower incisor to the kidneys, the

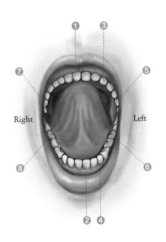

❶ The upper incisor connects to the heart
❷ The lower incisor connects to the kidneys
❸ The upper canine and premolar connect to the stomach
❹ The lower canine and premolar connect to the spleen
❺ The upper left molar connects to the gallbladder
❻ The lower left molar connects to the liver
❼ The upper right molar connects to the large intestine
❽ The lower right molar connects to the lungs

The distribution of teeth and the corresponding viscera.

upper canine and premolar to the stomach, the lower canine and premolar to the spleen, the upper left molar to the gallbladder, the lower left molar to the liver, the upper right molar to the large intestine, and the lower right molar to the lungs. See the illustration on page 63.

Human teeth can reflect what is going on with the internal organs in the human body. Teeth are a relatively independent part of the human body, so when a tooth aches, the pathological change of an internal organ can be directly determined from that tooth alone.

Teeth grinding. The upper and lower teeth grind against each other and make a "clicking" sound. Teeth grinding at night can cause excessive wear of children's teeth and a dysfunction of the temporomandibular joints. There are several factors contributing to teeth grinding.

Emotional factors include excessive fatigue and overstressed.

Systemic factors include parasite infection, gastrointestinal disorders and malnutrition.

Abnormal occlusion between upper and lower teeth. Abnormal occlusion leading to a dysfunction of the temporomandibular joints.

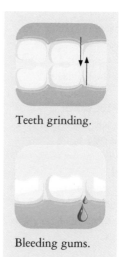

Teeth grinding.

Bleeding gums.

Bleeding gums. Blood oozing out between teeth or from gum lines is often a manifestation of fire in the body. For example, stomach fire and excess fire due to kidney deficiency can all result in gum bleeding. Gum inflammation is another cause for bleeding. Bleeding gums can also be a prominent symptom of scurvy.

Heavy bleeding accompanied by bad breath indicates excessive fire in the gastrointestinal system.

Pale red blood, accompanied by rotting gums indicates deficient fire in the stomach.

Pale red blood, accompanied by

loosening of teeth indicates hyperactive fire due to deficiency of the kidney.

Red and swelling gums, the edge of the gum turning ulcerous indicates gingivitis.

Gum bleeding, accompanied by loosening of the teeth indicates a sign of scurvy.

Loosening of the teeth. Often seen in the elderly. The Yangming meridian of the hand passes through the lower tooth bed, while the Yangming meridian of the foot passes through the upper tooth bed. Teeth are considered the remnants of bones and rely on the gums for nourishment. It is not hard to see how closely the loosening of the teeth is related to the Yangming meridian of the hand and foot, as well as the kidneys.

Loosening of the teeth, red and swelling gums indicate overactive heat blocking Yangming meridians.

Loosening of teeth, dizziness and tinnitus and hair loss indicate deficiency of kidney *yin*.

Loosening of teeth, sore lower back and difficulty emptying bladder indicate deficiency of kidney *qi*.

Gum inflammation, too much tartar, with periodontal pockets are caused by poor mouth hygiene.

Burnt black teeth. The teeth are dry with a lusterless black tinge. Often seen in patients with febrile illnesses and depletion of *yin* due to extreme heat. It is often suggestive of a poor prognosis.

Burnt black teeth, dry mouth and dry tongue indicate hyperactivity of heat in the lower burner.

Burnt black teeth, soiled, accompanied by dry throat and thirst, restlessness, and insomnia indicates depletion of *yin* due to stomach heat.

Yellowish black teeth, dry, accompanied by shaky teeth roots, sore and weak lower back and knees, hair loss indicates

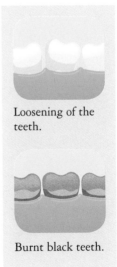

Loosening of the teeth.

Burnt black teeth.

insufficiency of kidney essence and wind-cold invading the meridian.

Tips for Caring for Your Teeth

The teeth are used to break down food and assist speaking. It is important to have a set of healthy teeth. Rinse your mouth after each meal to remove food residue between the teeth. Brush your teeth before going to bed, as germs tend to grow when saliva secretion is limited during sleep. Eat more vegetables high in water and fiber, which help clean the teeth. Regular check-ups of the teeth will help prevent dental diseases. A yearly check-up is recommended for adults.

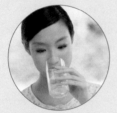

Rinse your mouth after each meal.

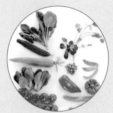

Eat more vegetables.

Chapter Three
Diagnosis and Treatment of Common Ailments

In modern society people are living a fast-paced life. They are so busy with their work that they have little time for rest. They have developed bad eating habits and are confronted with greater stress and pressure. As a result, many people are not in an optimal state of health. If we take some time to observe our bodies regularly, learn some methods of self-examination and self-treatment, and if problems can be discovered and treated early, we will be able to maintain good health. This chapter explains in detail the diagnostic face reading methods that can help detect nearly 40 common ailments and introduces related TCM therapies and daily care. The book's rich content will help readers self-examine and diagnose their own health problems and take good care of themselves. (Please note: For moxibustion treatments, pictures in this chapter illustrate the operation by showing a person with clothes on. In practice, however, readers should do moxibustion without clothing. All the acupoints for the Therapeutic Methods sections are illustrated, and you can also find the detailed description of their location in the Appendices.)

1. Common Cold

Known in modern Western medicine as acute infection of the upper respiratory tract, the common cold occurs year round, most commonly in winter and spring. TCM teaches that evil toxins enter the body through the mouth, nose, and skin, triggering the onset of the common cold. The common cold

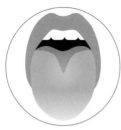

Patients can have thin and yellow tongue coating.

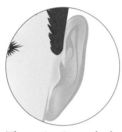

The patient's ears look red and feel warm.

typically runs a short course, from three to seven days, then the patient recovers.

The clinical manifestations are primarily stuffy or runny nose, sneezing, chills, fever, headache, and general body aches. Some patients may also show problems with the spleen and stomach, exhibiting symptoms of chest tightness, nausea, vomiting, loss of appetite, and loose stool. Colds are mostly caused by the invasion of wind pathogens, resulting in the functional imbalance of the lungs.

Face Reading

Cold of a wind-heat type, caused by the invasion of wind-heat pathogens through the surface of the human body, exhibits symptoms such as thin, yellow tongue coating with a slimy texture and the tip of the tongue turning slightly red. Cold of a wind-cold type, often occurring in winter or early spring and caused by the invasion of wind-cold pathogens, will have symptoms including a white tongue coating, accompanied by a pale complexion, severe chills, headache, and a runny or stuffy nose. If the patient's ears look red and feel warm, it may be a sign of influenza.

Therapeutic Methods

When infected with colds, you should strive for a balanced daily routine of work and rest, and a proper diet. Open windows for ventilation and avoid getting too cold. Avoid going to public places to reduce the chances of infection.

Dietary advice: Drink plenty of water, eat foods that are light and easy to digest, and avoid foods that are spicy, pungent, oily and highly sweet.

Exercise: Exercise regularly to improve your physical constitution as a means of preventing the onset of the common cold. Once infected, however, do not exercise vigorously, because your immune system is weak at this time and too much exercise will worsen the symptoms. Adequate bed rest is recommended.

Emotional adjustment: Maintain a balanced state of mind and avoid mood swings. Do not feel upset because of the cold. A bad mood is not conducive to recovery.

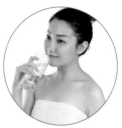

Drinking plenty of water can boost the recovery of common cold.

Moxibustion: When you have a cold and feel cold in the extremities, cold pain in the shoulders and back, or have general weakness in the body, a mild-warm moxibustion[1] treatment at the Dazhui point will improve the symptoms. Use a moxa stick to heat the Dazhui point for 10 minutes, once or twice daily. Hold the burning end of the moxa stick at a certain distance away from the skin so the patient feels the warmth without being burned. This helps dispel wind and clear cold, thereby effectively improving the body's immune system and relieving the symptoms of the cold.

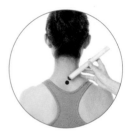

Dazhui point.

Massage: In the early stage of the onset, massaging certain acupoints

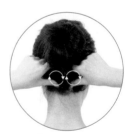

Fengchi points.

can improve the symptoms. Pressing the Fengchi, Taiyang, Yingxiang, Dazhui, and Zusanli points will dispel wind and clear cold, strengthen the body's immune system, and prevent and treat a cold. Using the thumb or middle finger, press each

---

1 Mild-warm moxibustion. Ignite the end of the moxa stick and put it close to the acupoint at a proper distance so the patient feels the warmth without being burnt. This type of moxibustion usually lasts 10 to 15 minutes.

acupoint clockwise first for two minutes, then counterclockwise for another two minutes. Stop massaging until a soreness and distending pain appears in the acupoint. Do this three times every day.

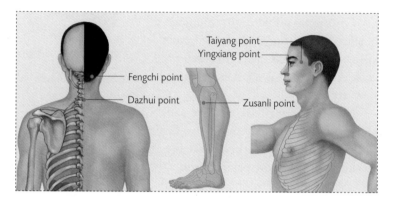

2. Chronic Bronchitis

Chronic bronchitis is a chronic non-specific inflammation of the trachea, bronchial mucosa, and surrounding tissues. The onset is slow and the course of the disease is long. There may be repeated episodes before the condition worsens. Chronic bronchitis typically lasts for three months each year and can go on for two consecutive years or more.

Common symptoms are repeated coughing, expectoration and shortness of breath, and sticky, white, foamy sputum. Western medicine attributes the onset of chronic bronchitis to two causes. The first is a compromised local immune system of the respiratory tract, resulting in the respiratory tract infections, and the second is the dysfunction of the autonomic nervous system that renders the respiratory tract easily irritated.

Face Reading
There are blood streaks on the tip of the nose and on both cheekbones, or dilated capillaries on the lung zone of the ears.

Part of the iris or the entire bulbar conjunctiva is covered with fatty substances that are yellow in color.

Therapeutic Methods

Patients suffering from chronic bronchitis should avoid catching colds. Exercise more to strengthen the body's resistance to diseases, consume a light diet, and quit smoking or consuming alcohol.

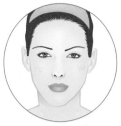

Red streaks on the tip of the nose and both cheekbones. Part of the iris is yellow.

Dietary advice: Your diet should be light and easy to digest, and make sure you take in plenty of protein by eating such food as eggs, lean meat, and milk. Avoid foods that are cold, raw, overly sweet, oily, and spicy.

Exercise: Do more physical exercise. Swimming is recommended in summer because swimming can not only improve the lung's function of *qi* exchange but also increase breathing capacity.

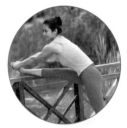

Exercise more to strengthen the body's resistance to the disease.

Emotional adjustment: Therapy for chronic bronchitis takes a long time. You must be patient once infected with the disease and remain calm and in a balanced state of mind. Family members should give the patient extra care. Harmful emotions should be alleviated in a timely manner.

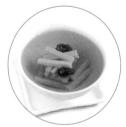

Pumpkin and red date soup.

Medicinal diet therapy: Consume pumpkin and red date soup. Mix 150 grams of pumpkin, two red dates, and some brown sugar. Remove the pumpkin skin and cut the flesh into strips, then cook them with the red dates to make the soup. This soup relieves exterior syndromes and ventilates the lungs. It is an effective supplementary treatment for chronic bronchitis.

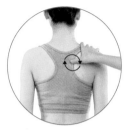

Feishu point.

Massage: Acupoints such as the Feishu, Shenshu, Huagai, Zhongfu, Chize, and Hegu all have the effect of relieving exterior syndromes and ventilating the lungs, replenishing the kidney to promote *yang*, dispersing the lungs to relieve coughing, and clearing lung heat. Continued massage treatment can relieve the symptoms of chronic bronchitis to a certain extent. Use your thumb, index finger, or middle finger to massage the acupoint, first clockwise for about two minutes, then counterclockwise for about two minutes. Stop when there is soreness and distending pain in the acupoint. Do this three times a day.

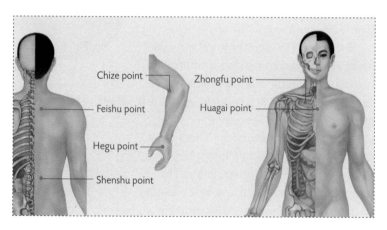

3. Pharyngitis

Pharyngitis refers to the inflammation of the mucous membrane and lymphatic tissue of the pharynx. According to the time of onset and different symptoms, it is divided into acute pharyngitis and chronic pharyngitis. The causes are mainly a disorderly lifestyle, the failure of defensive *qi* to protect the lungs, and wind-heat pathogens invading the throat.

Clinical manifestations include pharyngeal discomfort, the

sensation of an existent foreign body, pharyngeal secretions that are hard to spit out, sensations of itchiness, burning, dryness, or irritation of the pharynx, and occasional slight pain. Acute pharyngitis, which is often a viral or bacterial infection, is more common in winter and spring, while chronic pharyngitis results from repeated episodes of acute pharyngitis.

Face Reading

Sudden redness of both earlobes without stimulation indicates inflammation of the tonsils. If black spots appear on the earlobes, it may indicate chronic pharyngitis.

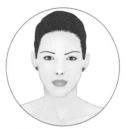

Black spots appear on the earlobes.

Therapeutic Methods

To treat pharyngitis, chronic pharyngitis in particular, patients should follow the principle of "thirty percent treatment and seventy percent daily care."

Dietary advice: Do not eat spicy, pungent, fried, and pickled foods, quit smoking and consuming alcohol, and eat foods rich in vitamins and those that aid in clearing heat, soothing the pharynx, and relieving thirst, such as kiwi fruit and watermelon.

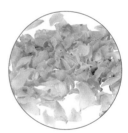

Lily bulbs.

Exercise: Get plenty of exercise to strengthen the body's resistance, but do it on warm afternoons when the temperature has gone up and the dust concentration has been reduced.

Lifestyle: Make sure that you get plenty of sleep, avoid late nights, and speak less. Brush your teeth in the morning and at night to keep your oral cavity clean.

Medicinal diet therapy: Consume

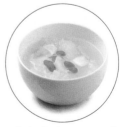

Lily bulb, banana, and white fungus soup.

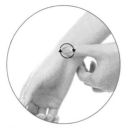

Jingqu point.

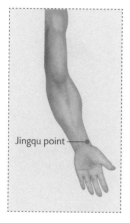

Jingqu point

lily bulb, banana, and white fungus soup. Lily bulbs and dried white fungus 30 g each, two bananas, Chinese wolfberries (*goji* berries), and rock sugar. Peel the banana skin and cook the flesh in water with lily bulbs, soaked white fungus and Chinese wolfberries. Add the rock sugar to improve the taste when the soup is ready. This soup nourishes the lungs and is suitable for patients with pharyngitis.

Massage: Massaging the Jingqu point helps alleviate coughing, pharyngitis, and sore throat. In modern medicine, this massage method can be used in the prevention of respiratory diseases such as bronchitis, pneumonia, pharyngitis, and tonsillitis. Use the pad of the middle finger to knead the Jingqu point for three minutes three times a day.

4. Tonsillitis

Tonsillitis is a non-specific acute inflammation of the palatine tonsils. It is often accompanied by a degree of acute inflammation of the pharyngeal mucosa and pharyngeal lymphatic tissue.

At the acute onset, the patient feels severe pain in the pharynx, radiating to the ear. The pain is aggravated when swallowing. The illness is often accompanied by a high grade fever, aversion to cold, and head and torso aches. If the illness lasts a long time, the patient may have a dry, itchy throat, difficulty swallowing, the sensation of a foreign body lodged in the throat, or a recurrent sore throat and fever. Chronic tonsillitis is mostly the result of delayed treatment of acute tonsillitis.

Face Reading

If earlobes turn red within a short period of time, it indicates an acute attack of chronic tonsillitis. The tongue manifests redness, a thin, yellow tongue coating, with a dry, painful throat, difficulty swallowing, fever, and cough.

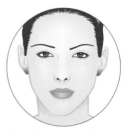

Earlobes turn red.

Therapeutic Methods

Consume a light diet, and eat foods that clear away heat and sooth the pharynx. Avoid pungent, irritating, raw, and cold foods, and avoid smoking and alcohol. Maintain oral hygiene by gargling with light salty water after meals to reduce the risk of oral bacterial infections.

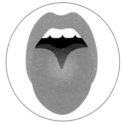

The tongue manifests redness, a thin, yellow tongue coating.

   Massage: The Kongzui point can assist with the treatment of tonsillitis. Use the pad of your thumb to massage the Kongzui point for three minutes, three times a day. Perseverance in massaging this point can dispel lung heat, help lung *qi* descend, and clear orifice collaterals, eliminating swelling, reducing pain, stimulating sound, and clearing the throat.

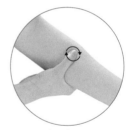

Kongzui point.

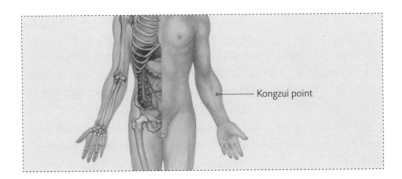

Kongzui point

5. Pulmonary Emphysema

Pulmonary emphysema refers to a pathological condition in which the distal end of the bronchioles (including respiratory bronchioles, alveolar ducts, alveolar sacs, and alveoli) are enlarged, accompanied by destructive changes in the cavity wall.

Common symptoms are fullness of the chest, oppression in the chest, as if it is blocked, coughing and panting, copious sputum, irritability, palpitations, and other similar symptoms. The condition is characterized by panting, coughing, phlegm, and distension, and it is mostly seen in the elderly, who often experience the onset triggered by external factors, though cold is the main culprit. Overexertion, anger, and blistering heat can also be triggers. Smoking, infection, and air pollution are also potential contributors to the onset of pulmonary emphysema.

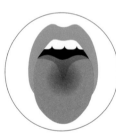

Dark purple tongue texture, greasy or turbid coating.

Face Reading
Dark purple tongue texture, greasy or turbid coating. The symptoms are coughing, copious foamy white sputum, wheezing, panting, difficulty lying flat, and chest fullness and compression.

Therapeutic Methods
Patients with pulmonary emphysema should quit smoking and keep warm to avoid catching colds and the common cold. Avoid pungent, greasy, and gas-causing foods. Keep your living environment clean, and eliminate or avoid factors that might affect the respiratory tract, such as smoke and dust.

Massage: Use your thumb to press-knead the Chize point for three minutes, until a distension is produced, once daily.

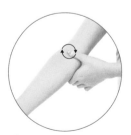

Chize point.

The Chize point is ideal for treating lung diseases because it has the function of replenishing the lung *qi* and nourishing the lung *yin*.

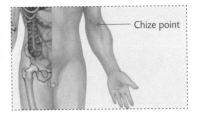

Chize point

6. Tuberculosis

Pulmonary tuberculosis is a chronic infectious disease resulting from a lung infection with mycobacterium tuberculosis. When the human body is infected with mycobacterium tuberculosis, he or she may not necessarily have an immediate onset. The onset only starts when the body's resistance is compromised or a cell-mediated allergic reaction increases.

The early symptoms include cough, coughing up phlegm, chest pain, hot flashes, night sweats, and gradual weight loss or loss of strength. In the later stage, the patient may cough up blood. Pulmonary tuberculosis is a result of two factors, internal and external. The external cause is that the lungs are infected with tuberculosis bacteria, and the internal cause is the weakening of the body's vital *qi*, leading to a decline in the body's resistance.

Face Reading

Pale complexions and flushed cheeks, as if rouged. On the ear's lung zone are red petechiae or small nodules the size of millet grains, which are signs of tuberculosis.

Therapeutic Methods

Tuberculosis is a chronic disease. Appropriate dietary habits and daily care are very helpful to the patient's recovery.

Dietary advice: As tuberculosis is also known as consumption, patients are advised to have a diet with foods high in

Flushed cheeks and small nodules in the ear.

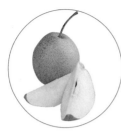

Pears can nourish the lungs and dispel phlegm.

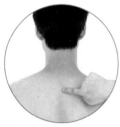

Shenzhu point.

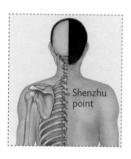

Shenzhu point

protein, calories, and vitamins and low in fat, with a reasonable combination of meat and vegetables. Pears, which can nourish the lungs and dispel phlegm, are a good ingredient for soup or porridge.

Exercise: Do low intensity exercises such as walking and yoga to enhance the respiratory circulation function, promote air exchange, and enhance the body's immunity.

Emotional adjustment: Tuberculosis patients should maintain an optimistic attitude. If they develop a negative attitude, become paranoid, fearful, and pessimistic, their condition will become worse.

Massage: Massaging the Shenzhu point, which connects to the lungs and are responsible for *qi*, is effective in treating such diseases as asthma, coughs and tuberculosis. Press the Shenzhu point with the pad of the index finger for one to three minutes, once daily. Massaging it long-term has the effect of replenishing *qi* to dispel evil, strengthening the body's resistance, and effectively improving the condition.

7. Chronic Gastritis

Chronic gastritis refers to a host of chronic gastric mucosal inflammations stemming from various causes. A common disease, it has the highest incidence among various gastric diseases.

Most patients are asymptomatic or experience varying degrees of indigestion, such as a dull pain in the upper abdomen, loss of appetite, abdominal fullness, or acid reflux. The main causes of chronic gastritis are long-term use of foods or drugs that are irritating to the gastric mucosa, excessive drinking, smoking, irregular eating habits, and intake of foods that are too cold or hot.

Face Reading
There are capillaries in the eyes moving towards the iris and several red patches on the tongue surface, and shiny dots or patches with a red tinge in the stomach zone of the ears.

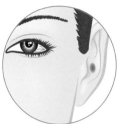

Capillaries in the eyes and shiny dots or patches in the ear.

Therapeutic Methods
Patients with chronic gastritis should exercise frequently and give attention to their diet to avoid upsetting the stomach.

Dietary advice: Consume a light diet, eat less fatty, sweet, greasy, spicy, and pungent foods. Drink less alcohol and less strong tea. Avoid consuming foods at extreme temperatures. Cold foods, such as ice cream, can irritate the stomach, and aggravate the symptoms, and are thus not recommended.

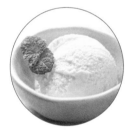

Ice cream can irritate the stomach.

Exercise: Do not engage in vigorous activities immediately after a meal, as it will cause indigestion. Rest for an hour after a meal before you exercise.

Emotional adjustment: Human emotions are closely related to the secretion of gastric acid and digestion. When your mood is low, even a delicious meal will taste as bland as wax. It is best to stay positive and relaxed at meal times.

Medicinal diet therapy: Codonopsis (*dang shen*) and red date tea. Codonopsis

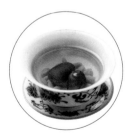

Codonopsis and red date tea.

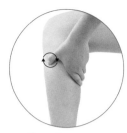

Zusanli point.

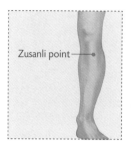

Zusanli point

15 g, 10 red dates, dried orange peel 3 g. Decoct these herbs to make a tea. Drink the tea twice a day for seven days as one course of treatment. This tea can nourish the spleen, replenish the stomach, reduce inflammation, and effectively improve the symptoms of chronic gastritis.

Massage: Massage the Zusanli point to replenish the spleen and stomach, regulate *qi* and blood, and improve deficiencies and weaknesses. This acupoint is mainly used to treat stomach diseases. Use your finger to press-knead the Zusanli point 50 times clockwise and 50 times counterclockwise, three times a day, until the skin feels distension.

8. Gastric and Duodenal Ulcers

This disease results from the decreased protective function of the local mucosa of the stomach and duodenum leading to its failure to balance the acidic gastric juices that aid digestion.

Clinically, the disease features a chronic process, periodic attacks, and rhythmicity of symptoms. The main symptoms are upper abdominal pain, nausea, vomiting, acid reflux, salivating, abdominal fullness, and constipation. Triggers include mood swings, unhealthy lifestyle habits, and side effects from drugs.

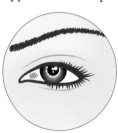

Reticular hyperplasia of the lower eyelid conjunctiva and bulbar conjunctival blood vessels.

Face Reading

Reticular hyperplasia of the lower eyelid conjunctiva and bulbar conjunctival blood vessels suggest pathological changes in the stomach and duodenum. Patients with gastric ulcers often have a thick yellow tongue coating and a red tongue texture, while those with duodenum ulcers mostly have a smooth tongue surface with no coating, or a thin layer of white coating, and their tongue is light or light red.

Therapeutic Methods

Consume a regular diet, avoid overeating, refrain from foods that are too sweet, too sour, too salty, and too hot, and foods that are raw, cold, hard, spicy, or pungent, because such foods tend to irritate the stomach. Eat more easily digestible foods.

Massage: Press-knead the Hegu point with your thumb for three minutes, three times a day. Press-knead until a distension is produced. The Hegu point is effective for diseases of the digestive system. Frequent massaging of this point can clear away heat and eliminate fire, and effectively relieve the symptoms of gastric and duodenal ulcers.

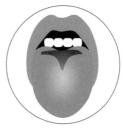

A thick yellow tongue coating and a red tongue texture.

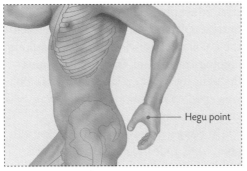

Hegu point

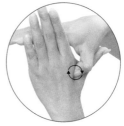

Hegu point.

9. Gastroptosis

Gastroptosis refers to a condition in which the lower edge of the stomach reaches the pelvic cavity when you are in the standing position, and the lowest point of the arc of the gastric minor curve drops below the inter-crestal line of the crista iliac. This is the result of a long-term eating disorder or excessive fatigue, which leads to the sinking of middle qi[1] and the failure to regulate the rise and fall of the stomach qi.

Most patients with mild gastroptosis are asymptomatic. Those with evident gastroptosis often have symptoms such as insufficient gastrointestinal energy and indigestion. Gastroptosis occurs when the diaphragm is unable to support the stomach, leading to the hypofunction and relaxation of the liver and stomach and diaphragmatic gastric ligaments. As a result there is a decrease in intra-abdominal pressure and the relaxation of the abdominal muscles. Other factors, such as body shape or physical constitution, render the stomach shape like a fish hook.

Face Reading

Oval-shaped chloasma on the bridge of the nose are a sign of gastriptosis. Several black spots appearing on the cheekbone area and around the eyes also suggest gastriptosis.

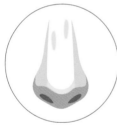

Oval-shaped chloasma on the bridge of the nose.

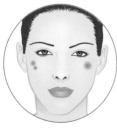

Several black spots appearing on the cheekbone area.

Therapeutic Methods

The key to alleviating gastroptosis is to strengthen physical fitness, stick to a high nutrition diet, and exercise to strengthen the abdominal muscles, including walking, jogging, and tai chi. Eat small but more frequent meals, chew slowly to break up your food more thoroughly, and avoid raw and cold foods.

Massage: Press-knead the Zhongwan point with your finger for about three minutes, three times a day. This soothes the liver and stomach, stopping pain and vomiting. Stack the palm of your left hand on the back of your right hand, attach the base of your right palm to your upper abdomen, massage your abdomen clockwise for three minutes, three times a day. This helps loosen your chest, regulate qi, and replenish the spleen and stomach.

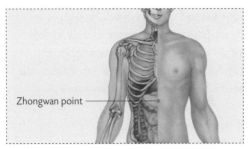

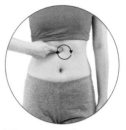

Zhongwan point.

10. Constipation

Constipation is not a disease in itself, but a symptom of other diseases. When abnormalities occur in the function of the large intestine, it can lead to constipation, a prolonged defecation cycle, or dry feces, making it difficult to defecate.

The onset of constipation is slow, and the condition is characterized as the process of a chronic disease. It is often accompanied by symptoms such as abdominal distension, abdominal pain, dizziness, bad breath, and hemorrhoids. There are many causes of constipation, but it is mainly related to factors such as an improper diet, a sedentary lifestyle, too little food intake, a lack of water, overeating foods that are pungent or strong in taste, block of *qi* movement, malnutrition, or an imbalance of the viscera.

Face Reading

If there are corrugated dark blood vessels in the inner canthus

---

1 Sinking of middle *qi*. Middle-*qi* refers to the spleen and stomach *qi*. When spleen *qi* deficiency occurs, its holding power declines and sinking happens instead. Its clinical manifestations are abdominal heaviness and distension, which worsens after meals, frequent bowel movements, heaviness and distention in the anus, prolonged diarrhea and dysentery, prolapse of the anus, prolapse of the uterus, or turbid urine. These symptoms are often accompanied by a general malaise, aversion to talking due to *qi* deficiency, low and feeble voice, lightheadedness and vertigo, shrunken physical shape, loss of appetite, and loose stool.

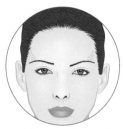

Visible veins above the temples.

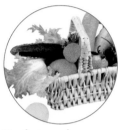

Eat fruits and vegetables that are rich in fiber to aid in intestine movement.

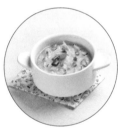

Chinese angelica and arborvilae seeds congee.

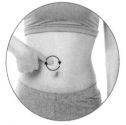

Shangqu point.

that extend to the cornea, it suggests constipation. If there are clearly visible veins above the temples resembling earthworm masses, this is most often the result of long-term constipation.

Therapeutic Methods

Constipation treatment focuses on lubricating the intestine and clearing heat. You should not only maintain good dietary habits, but also make proper adjustments in your lifestyle.

Dietary advice: Eat fruits and vegetables that are rich in fiber to aid in intestine movement. Eat foods high in pectin, such as bananas and carrots, to lubricate the intestine and make defecation easier.

Exercise: Run for an hour each day or do squats often. These are conducive to restoring your defecation reflex.

Emotional adjustment: Maintain a peaceful state of mind and be upbeat, avoid getting angry, and reduce your level of anxiety and stress.

Medicinal diet therapy: Chinese angelica (*dang gui*) and arborvilae seeds (*bai zi ren*) congee. Chinese angelica 20 g, Chinese arborvilae seeds 15 g, glutenous rice 50 g, Chinese wolfberries, and chopped green onions. Wash the Chinese angelica and arborvilae seeds, soak to soften the Chinese wolfberries, and add them with the glutenous rice to the pot, then cook to make a congee. Add the Chinese wolfberries and cook until the congee is ready. Finally, sprinkle the chopped green onions on top, and the congee is ready. This congee has the function of lubricating the intestine and loosening the bowels to relieve constipation.

Massage: Massage the Shangqu point, which has the effect of transporting and transforming water and dampness and clearing heat. Massage the Shangqu point with your thumb, press-kneading for three minutes until a distension is felt, three times a day. This has a significant alleviating effect for symptoms such as abdominal pain and constipation.

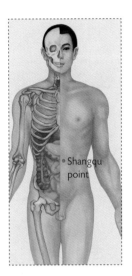

Shangqu point

11. Enteritis

Enteritis is a disease caused by microbial infections from bacteria and viruses. It is a common disease. It can be classified according to the course of the disease into acute enteritis and chronic enteritis.

The main symptoms of acute enteritis are nausea, vomiting, and diarrhea. The main symptoms of chronic enteritis are long-term repeated episodes of abdominal pain, diarrhea, and indigestion. Acute enteritis is mostly a result of an improper diet, cold attacking the abdomen, or eating rotten or contaminated food. Chronic enteritis is mostly caused by chronic intestinal infections or inflammatory diseases.

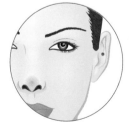

Face Reading
Redness of the nostrils and a blue tip of the nose may indicate enteritis and spots or flaky congestions in the large and small intestine zones of the ears, which are rosy, shiny, and seborrheic are signs of acute diarrhea.

Redness of the nostrils and a blue tip of the nose.

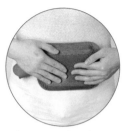

A hot water bottle can be used to warm the abdomen.

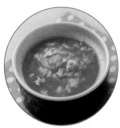

Lotus leaf and poria cocos porridge.

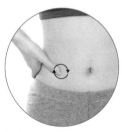

Daheng point.

Therapeutic Methods

Patients with enteritis should avoid catching cold and keep the abdomen warm. When attacked by cold, a hot water bottle can be used to warm the abdomen. Control your emotions, adjust your diet, stop smoking, and limit alcohol intake to prevent your stomach from irritation.

Dietary advice: Maintain a regular diet, and eat more easily digestible foods. Avoid foods that cause gas and upset stomach. Avoid pungent foods and those rich in crude fiber that are indigestible.

Exercise: Increase physical exercise to enhance the body's resistance. Choose sports that are suitable to you, such as running, walking, yoga, or ball games.

Emotional adjustment: Maintain a good mindset and avoid excessive mental stress. These methods are conducive to keeping the disease in check and preventing the recurrence of enteritis.

Medicinal diet therapy: Lotus leaf and poria cocos (*fu ling*) porridge. One piece of lotus leaf, poria cocos 30 g, short-grain rice 60 g. Decoct the lotus leaf and remove the residue, but keep the juice. Wash the short-grain rice, put it into the pot with poria cocos, add the decocted juice to the mix, and cook the porridge. This porridge can replenish *qi* and invigorate the spleen. It is suitable for patients with chronic enteritis caused by a spleen deficiency, and it relieves enteritis-induced diarrhea.

Massage: Massage the Daheng point, which has the function of removing dampness and dispelling stagnation, regulating *qi* and invigorating the spleen, clearing the intestines, and regulating the stomach. This is an acupoint mainly for gastrointestinal diseases. Using your thumb to press-knead the Daheng point for three minutes, three times a day. Press-knead until you feel the distension. Long-term massaging of this point can help remove intestinal waste and effectively alleviate the symptoms of enteritis.

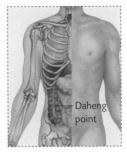

Daheng point

12. Fatty Liver

Fatty liver is caused by excessive buildup of fat in the liver cells. The fat content in a normal liver accounts for three to five percent of the liver. When the fat in the liver accounts for more than five percent, the liver is considered a fatty liver.

Fatty liver is characterized by mild to moderate liver dysfunction and hyperlipidemia. In mild cases, there are almost no symptoms, or only stiffness and distension in the liver area. In severe cases, however, patients will experience major symptoms such as pain, fatigue, indigestion, and swelling of the liver. Fatty liver can be a result of obesity, diabetes, drug poisoning, alcohol intoxication, viral hepatitis, and malnutrition.

Face Reading

The middle section of the bridge of the nose is the liver zone. If there are scattered yellow spots there, it may indicate a fatty liver. If the liver zone of the face is dark in color or has skin spots, you should attend to the fatty liver.

Therapeutic Methods

Set regular meal times and consume regular amounts of food. Do not overeat at dinner to control calorie intake. Eat whole grains, vegetables, fruits, and soy bean products. Control alcohol intake,

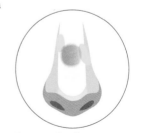

Scattered yellow spots or dark color on the bridge of the nose.

because alcohol abuse can seriously damage the liver and reduce its metabolic capacity.

Massage: The Yanglingquan is the main point for the treatment of fatty liver. Use your thumb to press-knead the Yanglingquan point 30 to 50 times once a day until

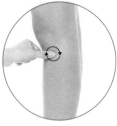

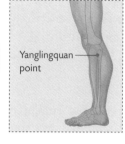

Yanglingquan point

distension is generated. Long-term massage treatment works very well to alleviate the symptoms of fatty liver.

Yanglingquan point.

13. Chronic Hepatitis

Chronic hepatitis is a chronic inflammatory disease of the liver caused by many factors, and the course of the disease lasts generally more than six months. Most of the hepatitis you will hear discussed refers to viral hepatitis caused by two types of hepatitis viruses, A and B.

Common symptoms are fatigue and stomach discomfort, which are easily overlooked. The manifestations are primarily extreme fatigue, nausea, vomiting, abdominal bloating, jaundice, and loss of appetite. Some patients have scleral or

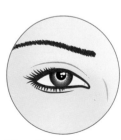

The whites of the eyes are yellow and the iris is deformed and appears dark brown.

skin infections. The pathogen is often related to factors such as viral infection, decreased autoimmunity, the influence of drugs and alcohol, and abnormal metabolism.

Face Reading

When the whites of the eyes are yellow, it suggests jaundice hepatitis. When the iris is deformed and appears dark brown, it suggests chronic hepatitis.

Therapeutic Methods

Patients with chronic hepatitis should be quarantined, stop drinking alcohol, and quit smoking to protect the liver. Periodic rest should be incorporated at work to avoid excessive fatigue.

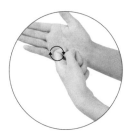

Massage the liver zone on the hands.

Dietary advice: Eat foods high in protein and vitamins, and avoid excessive intake of carbohydrates to prevent fatty liver. All alcoholic beverages are to be strictly eliminated.

Exercise: Work and rest should be properly balanced. After the liver function improves, you can do some exercise, such as walking. Appropriate amounts of exercise are conducive to physical recovery.

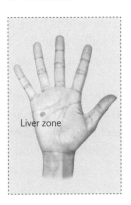

Liver zone

Emotional adjustment: If patients with chronic hepatitis feel depressed, their condition will worsen. It is imperative to maintain a good mood so the liver can be nourished and protected, which is ultimately conducive to recovery.

Massage: Massage the liver zone on the hands, stimulating the liver. This will improve the symptoms of chronic hepatitis. Bend the index finger and push-press the liver zone for three to five minutes once daily.

14. Cholecystitis and Gallstones

Cholecystitis is an inflammatory disease of the gallbladder that has various causes, which is classified into acute and chronic cholecystitis. Gallstones result from certain changes in the composition of bile, leaving the cholesterol to harden in the bile and form stones.

The onset of acute cholecystitis is manifested as sudden pain of the upper right abdomen, a feverish sensation, chills, nausea, and vomiting. The symptoms of gallstones are episodes of abdominal pain and acute inflammation. Cholecystitis is caused by bacterial infections in the gallbladder or roundworms in the intestine. Gallstones are caused by the gradual calcification of cholesterol in the bile.

Face Reading

When the nose looks like a gallbladder in shape, and light yellow spots appear on both sides of the nose, it often suggests diseases associated with the gallbladder. When nodules the size of millet grains appear in the pancreatic and gallbladder zones of the ear, it suggests gallstones.

Therapeutic Methods

Daily care is crucial to the recovery of patients with cholecystitis and gallstones. Consume a proper diet and balance the emotions to protect liver and gallbladder.

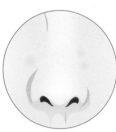

Light yellow spots appear on both sides of the nose.

Dietary advice: Adjust your diet and control the intake of foods high in fat and cholesterol, such as fatty meat, animal offal, and egg yolks. Do not drink alcohol, and avoid pungent and fried foods.

Exercise: People who work indoors and people with obesity should do more outdoor activities, such as running, walking, and playing ball games.

Emotional adjustment: Emotional disorders can easily lead to neurological disorders and cholestasis. It is important to be optimistic and keep an open mind, which is conducive to the improvement of the condition.

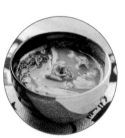

Corn silk and clam soup.

Medicinal diet therapy: Corn silk and clam soup. Corn silk 50 g, ginger 15 g, clam meat 150 g, and some salt. Wash and slice the clam meat and ginger, put the ingredients together with the corn silk in an earthenware pot. Add some water, simmer for an hour on low heat, and season with salt. The soup can clear away heat and invigorate the gallbladder, and is therefore suitable for people with cholecystitis and gallstones. Corn silk can accelerate bile excretion.

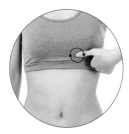

Qimen point.

Massage: The Qimen point has the effect of soothing the liver, promoting *qi*, clearing blood stasis, and resolving stagnation. It is mainly used to treat diseases such as cholecystitis and bloating in the sternum area. Use your thumb to press-knead the Qimen point for three to five minutes, once daily until a distension is produced.

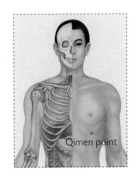

Qimen point

15. Hyperthyroidism

Hyperthyroidism is an endocrine disease caused by excessive secretion of the thyroid hormones as a result of a number of conditions. Pathologically, it is a diffuse disease.

Common symptoms of hyperthyroidism include increased appetite and defecation, an enlarged thyroid gland, anxiety and irritability, a bitter taste in mouth, a dry throat, mildly prominent eyes, sluggish eyelids, weight loss, and sweaty palms. The onset of hyperthyroidism often has certain triggers, of which the most common are infection, pneumonia, tonsillitis, pregnancy, and emotional trauma.

Face Reading

Facial manifestations of hyperthyroidism are a thick neck accompanied by a vascular murmur. Most patients also have symptoms such as bulging eyes, swollen eyelids, and vision loss.

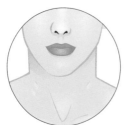

Thick neck.

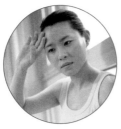

Patients with hyperthyroidism should rest and avoid excessive fatigue.

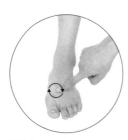

Taichong point.

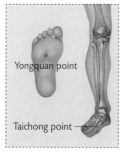

Yongquan point

Taichong point

Therapeutic Methods

Diet plays an especially important role in the treatment of hyperthyroidism. At the same time, increase your physical exercises and balance your mood. Patients with hyperthyroidism should rest and avoid excessive fatigue.

Dietary advice: Eat less pungent foods and more fresh fruits and vegetables. Maintain a high protein diet.

Exercise: Patients with hyperthyroidism should avoid strenuous exercise. The best exercise is yoga, which not only enhances physical fitness, but also regulates emotions.

Emotional adjustment: Patients with hyperthyroidism are prone to irritability, and long-term irritability can worsen the condition. It is important to regulate your emotions, and a good mood and balanced mental state will benefit recovery.

Massage: Massaging the Taichong point can clear away liver fire, dredge the liver, and regulate *qi*. It can also relieve hyperthyroidism caused by stagnation of liver *qi*. Massaging the Yongquan point can dispel heat and open the orifices, nourish *yin* and reduce fire, and alleviate symptoms such as irritability, aversion to heat, and excessive perspiration caused by hyperthyroidism. Press-knead the Taichong and Yongquan points with your thumb for one to three minutes, once daily.

16. Diabetes

Diabetes is a series of metabolic disorders caused by hypofunction of the pancreas, insufficient insulin secretion, or the body's inability to effectively use insulin. The disorders trigger metabolic failure to deal with things such as sugar, protein, fat, water, and electrolytes.

Typically, the clinical symptoms of diabetes are increased hunger, thirst, and urination and weight loss. Common symptoms also include dry mouth, and a bitter or peculiar taste in the mouth. The onset of diabetes may be related to factors such as heredity, lifestyle disorders, microbial infections, viruses, emotional stress, obesity, and age.

Face Reading
Small red dots are often seen on the whites of the eyes in patients with diabetes. The patient may look emaciated and have loose teeth that are frequently inflamed. They also feel numbness of the hands and feet and drowsiness. They experience a sudden rapid loss of vision and refractive errors. Diabetes patients in the middle and late stages have tongues that are stiff and inflexible. The tongue body is bulky and has teeth marks. The tongue is blue in color, with the front part being light blue. There are red prickles located on both sides of the tongue. The coating is thin and white, or there is little coating.

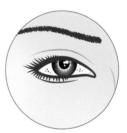

Small red dots on the whites of the eyes.

Therapeutic Methods
In addition to treatment by medication, patients with diabetes should be mindful of their diet, do proper exercises, maintain a healthy weight, and maintain a regular schedule of work and rest and a balanced

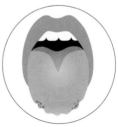

Teeth marks and red prickles on the tongue.

emotion. Diabetes patients should always pay attention to changes in their weight and keep it under control.

Dietary advice: The best dietary principle for diabetics is less oil, less salt, less sugar, and regular meals with regular amounts of food at fixed times. Limit the intake of staple foods and fats, and avoid sugary drinks, tobacco and alcohol, strong tea, and coffee.

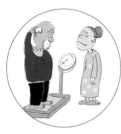

Diabetes patients should always pay attention to changes in their weight.

Exercise: Do appropriate amounts of aerobic exercises regularly and control your weight. Exercise should be done about an hour after a meal. Do not exercise while hungry.

Emotional adjustment: Patients should learn to control their emotions, avoid being too stressed, keep negative emotions in check, and maintain a peaceful state of mind.

Medicinal diet therapy: Salvia root (*dan shen*), soybeans, and pork rib soup. Soybeans 100 g, pork ribs 150 g, salvia root 10 g, some kohlrabi, ginger, and salt. Soak the soybeans in advance, wash and chop the ribs, shred the kohlrabi, and slice the ginger. Put all the ingredients in an

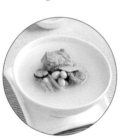

Salvia root, soybeans, and pork rib soup.

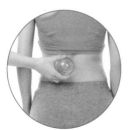

Shenshu point.

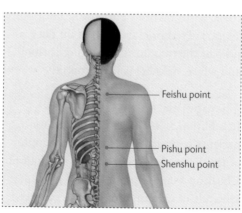

Feishu point

Pishu point

Shenshu point

earthenware pot, add some salt, and cook together until they are ready. This soup can invigorate the spleen and moisturize dryness.

Cupping: The Feishu point can increase thirst, the Pishu point can increase hunger, and the Shenshu point can increase urination. Cupping the above acupoints for five to ten minutes each, once a week.

17. Heart Disease

Heart disease is an umbrella term that includes such conditions as rheumatic heart disease, congenital heart disease, hypertension heart disease, coronary heart disease, and myocarditis. Common symptoms are palpitation, shortness of breath, coughing, coughing up blood, chest pain, edema, and abnormally little urination. There are two causes. The first is congenital, including heart defects developed while a fetus and pathogenic changes leading to changes in the tissues of the heart. The other is secondary, in which the heart has developed pathogens due to external impact or factors of internal mechanisms.

Face Reading
When the tip of the nose turns purple-blue or suddenly swells up, it indicates congenital heart disease. When the outer canthus of the eye has a large curved blood vessel that is dark in color, it indicates arrhythmia.

Therapeutic Methods
Patients with heart disease should take good care of their health on a day-to-day basis to protect and nourish their heart through proper diet, exercise, lifestyle, and balanced emotions.

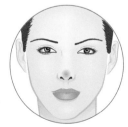

The tip of the nose turns purple-blue, and the outer canthus of the eye has curved blood vessels.

Dietary advice: Eat foods rich in dietary fiber to reduce the generation of cholesterol. Eat green leafy vegetables and supplement vitamins to promote

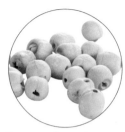

Lotus seeds can be eaten often by patients suffering from heart disease.

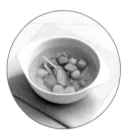

Lotus seeds, lily bulbs, and lean pork stew.

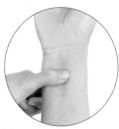

Neiguan point.

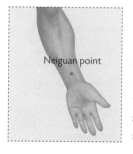

Neiguan point

blood circulation. Supplement with micro-elements. Lotus seeds, which contain liensinine that fights arrhythmia, can be eaten often by patients suffering from heart disease.

Exercise: Appropriate exercise can work to the benefit of your body and enhance your physical fitness. Choose low intensity exercises. Do not strain and put your body at risk.

Emotional adjustment: Maintain a regular schedule, cultivate a wide range of hobbies, get adequate amounts of sleep, and maintain balanced emotions. Keep your anxiety in check and prevent depression.

Medicinal diet therapy: Lotus seeds, lily bulbs, and lean pork stew. Lotus seeds and lily bulbs 10 g each, lean pork 200 g, and salt. Wash the lotus seeds and lily bulbs, add an appropriate amount of water, and cook for about 30 minutes. Wash the lean pork and cut into cubes. Add it into the pot and cook until well done, and add salt to taste. This soup can replenish the heart, calm the mind, and protect the heart.

Massage: Use your thumb to press the Neiguan point for three minutes, one to three times a day. This is helpful in relieving chest tightness and precordial discomfort, and in regulating the heart rate. Massaging your chest and patting the zone related to the heart is effective, to some extent, in eliminating chest tightness and pain.

18. Hypertension

Hypertension is a common medical condition primarily characterized by elevated systemic arterial blood pressure. It is generally believed that people under the age of 40 with a blood pressure higher than 140/90 mmHg when at rest are considered to have high blood pressure.

Elevated arterial blood pressure is the main clinical symptom. It can cause pathological changes in organs such as the blood vessels, brain, heart, and kidney. The main symptoms include headaches, dizziness, heaviness in the head, tinnitus, blurred vision, forgetfulness, inattention, insomnia, fatigue, numbness of the limbs, and palpitations. The pathogens may be related to genetics, high-salt diet, obesity, and alcoholism.

Face Reading

When the heart zone of the ear shows round white spots, it suggests primary hypertension. When the earlobe is round and thick and has a diagonal line or wrinkle, it indicates that the person has high blood pressure. Most patients have a red tongue, or their tongue sides are bright red, but a small number of patients may have pale red tongues, and some have purplish red tongues and teeth impressions on both sides, and the lingual frenulum on the sides of the tongue's underside appear like thick branches or bulging columns.

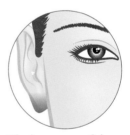

The heart zone of the ear shows round white spots, and the earlobe is round and thick.

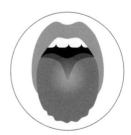

Teeth impressions on both sides of the tongue.

Therapeutic Methods

Changing unhealthy lifestyles is the key to the prevention of high blood pressure. Good care should be taken regarding dietary habits, exercise, and mood swings. Patients with hypertension should frequently check their blood pressure and be aware of the changes in their blood pressure readings at all time.

Dietary advice: Maintain a diet that is low in fat, salt, and calories. Eat frequently, but small meals. Eat foods high in calcium and potassium, but low in sodium, such as lettuce and milk.

Exercise: Exercise moderately and with appropriate methods, such as tai chi, yoga, jogging, and swimming. Do not exercise vigorously to avoid the risk of sudden increases in blood pressure, which is dangerous.

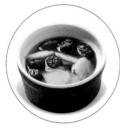

Celery and red dates soup.

Emotional adjustment: Maintain a positive state of mind. Maintain a balance between work and rest, keep your mind at ease, and avoid tension, irritability, and anxiety.

Medicinal diet therapy: Celery and red dates soup. Fresh celery stalks (lower end) 60 g and six to eight red dates. Wash the celery stalks and slice them, then wash the red dates. Put all the ingredients in a pot, add some water, and simmer on low heat for 30 minutes. This soup has the effect of lowering blood pressure and cholesterol. Celery lowers blood pressure.

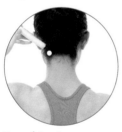

Fengchi point.

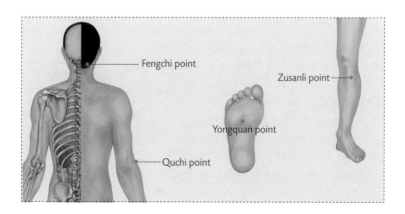

Moxibustion: The Fengchi and Quchi points can dispel wind and stabilize vertigo. The Yongquan point calms the liver, and the Zusanli point replenishes the spleen and promotes the harmony of *yin* and *yang*. Apply mild-warm moxibustion to these acupoints, each for about 15 minutes, once daily.

19. Hypotension

In general, when the arterial blood pressure of an adult's upper extremities is lower than 90/60 mmHg, it is considered hypotension. Most cases of hypotension are chronic, and the blood pressure is consistently below the normal range.

Hypotension can be classified into acute hypotension and chronic hypotension. The former includes symptoms such as dizziness, blackout, feeble extremities, cold sweats, palpitation, and scanty urination. In severe cases, the manifestations include syncope or shock. Chronic hypotension does not show obvious symptoms. Factors such as heart disease, peripheral blood vessel dilation, temporary blood loss in great amounts, and hypothyroidism can all cause hypotension.

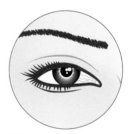

Wavy capillaries appear extending on the whites.

Face Reading
When wavy capillaries appear extending on the whites from the iris to the inner sides of the eyes flanking the bridge of the nose, it indicates hypotension. If small depressions appear in the earlobe, it suggests the risk of hypotension.

Therapeutic Methods
Maintain a regular work and rest schedule to ensure adequate sleep. Increase nutrition intake and eat nourishing foods such as longan, red dates, and lily bulbs. Frequent exercise can regulate the nervous

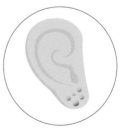

Small depressions appear in the earlobe.

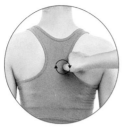

Xinshu point.

system and enhance the cardiovascular function.

Massage: Massaging certain acupoints can stimulate blood circulation, improve heart function, and invigorate physical function. Press-knead the Xinshu, Danzhong, and Guanyuan points with your thumb or middle finger, press-kneading each point for one to three minutes, three times a day. Apply force evenly and slowly. This massage will improve the symptoms of hypotension.

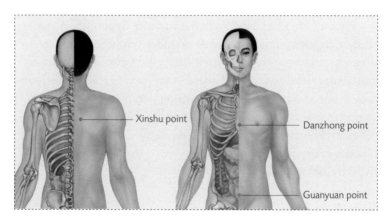

20. Dizziness

Dizziness is a general term for lightheadedness and vertigo. Lightheadedness refers to giddiness, blurred vision, or dim and fading vision. Vertigo refers to the sensation that the things you see are spinning, though they are not, or as if the world is moving and you are off balance. This condition can be classified as central or peripheral vertigo.

Dizziness is manifested as giddiness and blurred vision. In mild cases, just close your eyes and rest for a while, and you will be fine. In severe cases, there will be unsteadiness or even fainting, sometimes accompanied by nausea and vomiting.

TCM teaches that dizziness is mostly the result of a deficiency. *Yin* deficiency, insufficient blood, and damage of essence all contribute to various discomforts and cause dizziness. Other factors such as weakness of the spleen and stomach, phlegm-dampness obstructing the middle burner, and the imbalance of *yin* and *yang* in the body can also cause dizziness.

Face Reading

When there are spiral blood vessels above the inner canthus, with a large area of congestion in the corner of the eye, it usually indicates dizziness.

Therapeutic Methods

Move your neck frequently to prevent cervical vertigo. Dizziness is mostly triggered by the neck or head's movements. This is particularly evident during strenuous exercise. At the onset of dizziness, the patient can also experience nausea, vomiting, tinnitus, hearing impairment, and blurred vision. At the

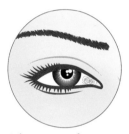

A large area of congestion in the corner of the eye.

onset of a dizziness episode, patients with mild symptoms can apply menthol balm to the temples to relieve headaches. Make sure to get adequate sleep and avoid anxiety and mental stress.

Massage: The Baihui point is closely connected with the brain and is the key point for regulating brain function. Frequent massage of the Baihui point can be a supplementary treatment for dizziness. Before going to sleep, sit straight and massage the Baihui point with your fingers, 100 times per session. Do this once daily, and stop massaging when a warm sensation is produced.

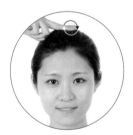

Baihui point.

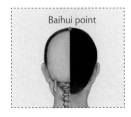

Baihui point

21. Insomnia

Insomnia is the inability to sleep normally, resulting in an unrefreshed state of mind during the day, unresponsiveness, and fatigue, which seriously affect one's daily life, work, and study.

Insomnia is manifested as difficulty falling asleep, difficulty staying asleep, and unsatisfying sleep, accompanied by symptoms such as fatigue, memory deterioration, slow response, difficulty concentrating, and headaches. TCM holds that the heart is in charge of the mind. Sleep problems belong in the jurisdiction of the heart. When you experience a deficiency of *qi* and blood, your heart is not nourished properly, leading to low spirits, stagnation of liver *qi*, and disorders of gastrointestinal function, all of which can cause obstruction of *qi* flow, which disturbs the mind and leads to insomnia.

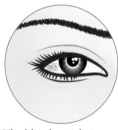

The blood vessels in the outer canthi of the eyes.

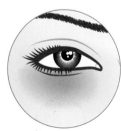

The skin under the eyelids turns bluish-black.

Face Reading

When the blood vessels in the outer canthi of the eyes are curved and the color grows darker, it is a sign of insomnia and dreaminess. For young people, the skin under the eyelids turning bluish-black is a sign of insomnia and dreaminess.

Therapeutic Methods

Develop healthy habits, go to bed at a fixed time, and avoid strong tea, coffee, and other stimulating beverages before bedtime. Maintain a light diet that is rich in protein and vitamins.

Massage: First, use your thumb to massage the Baihui point 50 times clockwise and 50 times counterclockwise, then press the Neiguan point with the tip of your thumb for three minutes. Finally, nip-press the Shaochong point with the tip of your thumb for one minute. This massage has the effect of replenishing and calming the heart and tranquilizing the mind to effectively alleviate the symptoms of insomnia. Do this every day before going to bed.

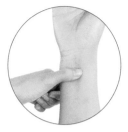

Neiguan point.

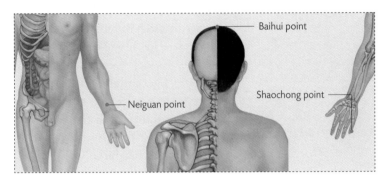

22. Tinnitus

Tinnitus refers to sound perception without any external stimuli. It is often a precursor to deafness and is caused by an auditory dysfunction.

The clinical manifestations of tinnitus are diverse. Tinnitus can happen in one ear or both ears, or it can occur in the head. The ringing can exist continuously or intermittently, in a variety of sound forms and varying pitches. Tinnitus can result from diseases of the auditory system, such as otitis media and otosclerosis. It can also be the result of systemic diseases, such as hypertension and arteriosclerosis.

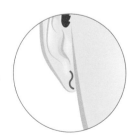

Face Reading

If a crease running diagonally upward

A crease running diagonally upward in the earlobe.

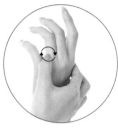

Yemen point.

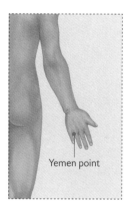

Yemen point

in the earlobe appears, or if the crease is above the earlobe, it is an indication of tinnitus.

Therapeutic Methods
People experiencing tinnitus often should take care of themselves on a daily basis. They should avoid loud noises, maintain a quiet living environment, and not use headphones to listen to music or for watching videos for a long time and at a high volume.

Massage: Every night before going to bed, massage the Yemen point for three to five minutes (with the finger of your choice), which can relieve symptoms such as headache, red eyes, earaches, loss of hearing, tinnitus, sore throat, and fever.

23. Headache

Headaches are a condition caused by external attacks and internal injury leading to twisted, spasmodic meridians or the failure to replenish the meridians blocking orifices. According to the International Headache Society, headaches are classified into primary headaches, secondary headaches, and other types of headaches.

The onset of headaches is often episodic, mostly on one side. It can happen from once a day to once several weeks, with each episode lasting from several hours to several days. With severe headaches, there are accompanying symptoms such as distension in the eyes and perspiration. The condition can be found at any age groups, but is more common in women. The onset is sudden and recurrent, and it can be induced by fatigue, insomnia, and emotional agitation.

Face Reading

Loss of eyebrow hair on one side is mostly caused by trigeminal neuralgia. The nose tilting to one side often indicates frequent headaches. Capillaries shaped like a match head in the white of the eye suggest headaches caused by traumatic head injury.

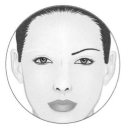

Loss of eyebrow hair on one side, and capillaries in the white of the eye.

Therapeutic Methods

When experiencing a headache, you can alleviate the symptoms by making adjustments in your lifestyle, such as diet, exercise, and mood control.

Dietary advice: Eat foods rich in magnesium, such as cashew nuts, almonds, or bananas, to relieve headache symptoms. Avoid alcohol and overconsumption of foods high in fat.

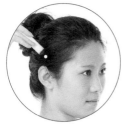

Shuaigu point.

Exercise: Exercise is one of the most effective ways to prevent headaches, because exercise can help alleviate tension and stress and relax the mind.

Emotional adjustment: Maintain a balanced emotional state. Listening to some quiet, relaxing music can regulate your mood. At the onset of a headache, close your eyes and meditate with the music on to divert your attention, which can relieve the headache for the moment.

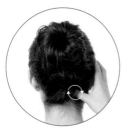

Fengchi point.

Moxibustion: Ignite a moxa stick, keep it three to five centimeters away from the Shuaigu point, and apply mild-warm moxibustion for about 10 minutes until a warm sensation is produced. Do it once daily. During the onset of a headache, moxibustion at the Shuaigu point can clear away heat and dispel wind to relieve headache symptoms.

Massage: Press-knead the Fengchi point 200 times with the

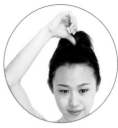

Baihui point.

pads of your thumbs. The intensity should increase gradually until a distension is produced. Do it once daily, or twice a day for severe headache patients. This massage can dispel wind and relieve the exterior to alleviate headaches as a result. Massaging the Baihui point at the onset of a headache is also effective for addressing headache symptoms.

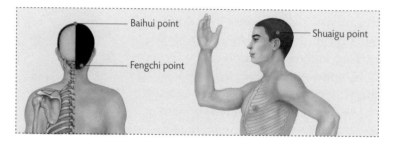

Baihui point

Fengchi point

Shuaigu point

24. Neurasthenia

Neurasthenia is a neurological condition caused by long-term excessive mental stress, excessive mental burdens or traumatic experiences leading to a host of clinical symptoms due to brain dysfunction.

Common clinical symptoms include emotional instability, pain due to tension, mental hyperactivity, fatigue, sleep disorders, and autonomic dysfunctions. Neurasthenia is a mental illness closely related to long-term depression, excessive worry and anxiety, and mental stress.

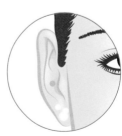

Circular folds in the ear and a flaky white patch at the anterior earlobe zone of the ear.

Face Reading
The tongue coating is pale, with teeth impressions on the tongue edge. In the ear's heart zone, circular folds can be seen,

and a flaky white patch can be seen at the anterior earlobe zone of the ear. The eyes usually have dark circles, the eyelids are puffy, and there are red blood streaks in the eyes.

Therapeutic Methods

Neurasthenia is mainly caused by one's mental state, so the patient should learn to self-regulate, avoid mental stress, and get enough rest. Soaking the feet in warm water before going to bed can promote blood circulation and help you sleep better.

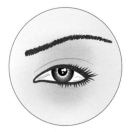

Dark circle under the eye.

Dietary advice: Include more foods that replenish the brain and clear the heart in your diet, such as crucian carp, lotus seeds, or longan. Do not drink strong tea or other caffeinated beverages at night.

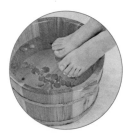

Soaking the feet in warm water before going to bed can help you sleep better.

Exercise: Do physical exercise to enhance your physical fitness, such as running, jumping aerobics, swimming, and playing badminton.

Emotional adjustment: Learn to self-adjust, confront whatever is unsatisfactory and stress-inducing in life with a positive attitude, cultivate an optimistic, open mindset, balance your work and rest, and do not overexert yourself.

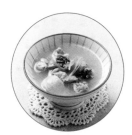

Chicken soup cooked with tall gastrodia tuber.

Medicinal diet therapy: Chicken soup cooked with tall gastrodia tuber (*tian ma*). One chicken, tall gastrodia tuber 15 g, dried shiitake mushrooms (after soaking) 50 g, chicken broth 500 ml, and some green onion and ginger. Wash and slice the tall gastrodia tuber and steam for 10 minutes. Cut the chicken into pieces, stir-fry with the green onion and ginger, add chicken broth, and bring to the boil, then turn to low heat and keep simmering for

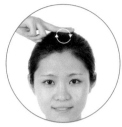

Baihui point.

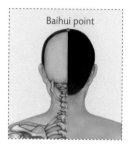

Baihui point

40 minutes. Add tall gastrodia tuber slices and simmer for five minutes, and the soup is ready. Tall gastrodia tuber, whose property is to calm the nerves and tranquilize the mind, helps relieve the symptoms of neurasthenia.

Massage: The Baihui point has the effect of clearing the orifices, refreshing the mind, soothing the liver, and dispelling wind. It mainly treats neurasthenia. Massaging the Baihui point for three to five minutes (with the finger of your choice) every day can relieve the symptoms of insomnia, dizziness, and headaches caused by neurasthenia.

25. Cerebral Arteriosclerosis

Cerebral arteriosclerosis is diffuse atherosclerosis of the cerebral arteries on the basis of systemic arteriosclerosis. It is characterized by the stenosis of the arteries, blockage of the small blood vessels, and reduced blood supply to the brain, all of which result in a series of neurological and mental symptoms.

Cerebral arteriosclerosis is clinically manifested as lightheadedness, headache, memory deterioration, mood swings, slow thinking, and sleep problems. The condition is mostly found in the middle-aged and the elderly. The pathogenesis is still unclear. In clinical practice, it has been found that it is more often a complication associated with patients with underlying conditions such as hypertension, hyperlipidemia, and diabetes.

Face Reading

Raised, twisted blue veins are seen on the temples. There are evident wrinkles on the earlobes and blood spots on the whites of the eyes. All these suggest higher than normal blood lipid levels, poor blood circulation, internal obstruction by turbid phlegm, and poor fluid flow in the body, resulting in a red tongue texture, dry and dull looking, and a thick yellow tongue coating.

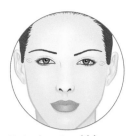

Raised, twisted blue veins on the temples.

Therapeutic Methods

Lead a regular life, consume an appropriate diet, persevere in physical exercise, and maintain emotional stability. Frequent massage for patients can relax the muscles and clear the meridians to promote blood circulation.

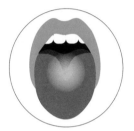

A red tongue texture and thick yellow tongue coating.

Dietary advice: The diet should be light and low in salt. Eat foods high in protein to avoid hardening of the blood vessels. Reduce meat intake. The elderly should avoid liquor.

Exercise: Do some exercise within your capacity, such as walking, gymnastics, tai chi, or traveling. These activities can facilitate the circulation of *qi* and blood and enhance your physical fitness.

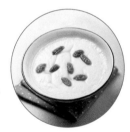

Chinese wolfberries and egg custard.

Emotional adjustment: Avoid mental stress and mood swings to reduce the occurrence of cerebral vasospasm. Make sure you maintain a balance between work and rest, lead a regular life, and maintain emotional stability.

Medicinal diet therapy: Chinese wolfberries and egg custard. Two eggs, Chinese wolfberries 6 g, and salt. Beat the eggs in a bowl and add the Chinese wolfberries. Add appropriate amount of water and salt and mix well. Steam the mixture in a pot. Chinese wolfberries have properties that fight aging, arteriosclerosis, and hyperlipidemia. This custard is especially suitable for the elderly.

Massage: Press the Neiguan point with the tip of your thumb for one to three minutes, three to five times a day, to replenish *qi* and promote blood circulation, remove blood stasis,

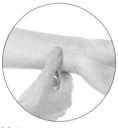

and dredge the collaterals to prevent arteriosclerosis. Press-knead the Shenmen point for one to two minutes with the pad of your thumb, three to five times a day. This massage calms the nerves and improves the symptoms of insomnia and headaches caused by cerebral arteriosclerosis.

Neiguan point.

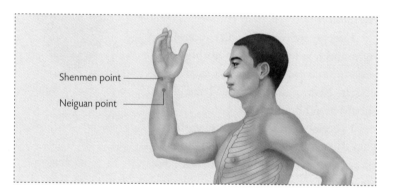

Shenmen point

Neiguan point

26. Cervical Spondylosis

Cervical spondylosis refers to the degeneration of the cervical intervertebral discs affecting the stability of the spine. Over time, this causes bone hyperplasia, which irritates or oppresses the spinal cord, nerve roots, vertebral arteries, and sympathetic nerves, leading to cervical spondylosis.

Common symptoms of cervical spondylosis include neck and back pain, weakness in the upper and lower limbs, numbness in the fingers, difficulty walking, lightheadedness, nausea, and vomiting. The causes include the wear and tear of the neck, cervical spine hyperplasia, incorrect posture, inflammation of the surrounding tissues, and neck trauma.

Face Reading

Raised nodules in the cervical vertebra zone of the ears is indicative of cervical spondylosis. Curved dark blood vessels on the upper eyeballs suggest neck pain.

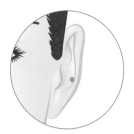

Raised nodules in the cervical vertebra zone of the ears.

Therapeutic Methods

Unhealthy lifestyle is one of the important causes of cervical spondylosis. Patients with cervical spondylosis can massage their shoulders and cervical spine often to relieve pain.

Dietary advice: Cervical spondylosis can be the result of vertebral hyperplasia and osteoporosis. Eat foods rich in calcium, protein, and vitamins.

Exercise: Participate in physical exercise that is appropriate to you. Correct bad sitting postures and do more exercises that require you to tilt your head upward. Move your shoulders often to improve the flexibility of your shoulder joints.

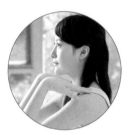

Patients with cervical spondylosis can massage their shoulders and cervical spine often.

Lifestyle: Avoid using a high pillow and sleep in an appropriate posture. Correct bad postures at work. Move the neck regularly, and avoid staying immobile in a sitting position for a prolonged period.

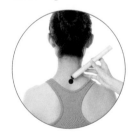

Dazhui point.

Moxibustion: Symptoms of cervical spondylosis can be relieved by moxibustion. Moxibustion of the Fengchi, Dazhui, Cervical Jiaji, and Jianjing points can dredge the meridians and dispel cold-dampness to facilitate the circulation of *qi* and blood. Each moxibustion session lasts about 15 minutes. Do this once daily.

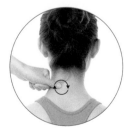

Bailao points.

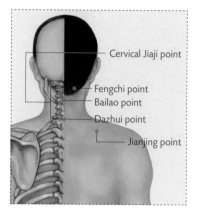

Cervical Jiaji point

Fengchi point
Bailao point
Dazhui point
Jianjing point

Massage: Frequent massaging of the Bailao points can relieve cervical fatigue. You can also interlock your fingers and place your hands behind the neck to rub the neck back and forth gently 50 times, until a warm sensation is produced in the neck. This will relax the cervical muscles. Massage three to five times a day.

27. Rheumatoid Arthritis

Rheumatoid arthritis is a common acute or chronic inflammation of connective tissues. This disease is very common, especially among the middle-aged and the elderly. Women are more likely than men to develop this disease.

The common symptoms of rheumatoid arthritis are symmetry and migratory pain in the joints and muscles, accompanied by signs of inflammation, such as redness, swelling, and a warm sensation. This disease is related to factors such as hemolytic streptococcus infection, humidity, cold, over-exertion, physical weakness, poor circulation of *qi* and blood, compromised immune system, injury, and malnutrition.

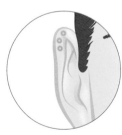

Small hard fleshy knots on the upper part of the helix.

Face Reading
A small hard fleshy knot on the upper part of the helix is called a "rheumatoid nodule." Clinically, it is found that patients having rheumatoid nodules often suffer from hyperostosis or arthritis.

Therapeutic Methods
If you have rheumatoid arthritis, you should treat it as soon as you

can. If untreated, it will cause great inconvenience.

Dietary advice: Eat more easily digestible, high-energy foods to enhance your physical resistance. Eat less pungent, cold, and greasy foods.

Exercise: During the remission period, do appropriate exercises to help improve the functions of joints, such as joint abduction and lifting. During an acute onset, lie in bed and avoid strenuous exercise.

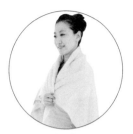

Dry your body immediately after a bath.

Lifestyle: Keep the joints warm. Avoid going out on cloudy days with overcast sky and on rainy days. Do not wear damp clothes. Dry your body immediately after a bath.

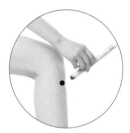

Zusanli point.

Moxibustion: Moxibustion can dispel wind, disperse cold, and eliminate dampness to relieve pain. Apply first to the Zusanli, Sanyinjiao, and Taixi points, which nourish the liver and kidney and replenish *qi* and blood. Then apply to the Ashi point[1] to dredge the collaterals and relieve pain. Finally, apply to the Dazhu and Yanglingquan points to relax the tendons and joints. Apply moxibustion to each point for about 15 minutes, once daily.

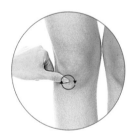

Dubi point.

Massage: Press-knead the Dubi, Xiyan and Quchi points with any finger for one to two minutes each, three to five

---

1 Ashi point. An Ashi point is not a specific acupoint, but a type of acupoint with no specific sites or designated names. The number of these points is uncertain, but they are chosen according to tender points, the location of pathological changes, or other response points for acupuncture purposes.

times daily until distension is produced on the skin. Regularly massaging these acupoints can dispel wind and dampness, disperse wind and cold, relax joints, clear the meridians, and relieve pain caused by rheumatoid arthritis.

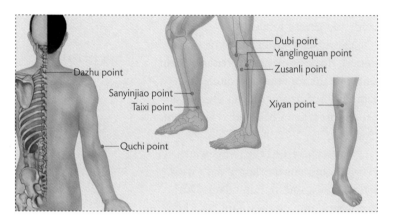

28. Lower Back Pain

This refers to pain in the lumbar spine or the side of the spine due to stagnant *qi* and blood movement or failure to replenish *qi* and blood in the lumbar region resulting from external invasion, internal damage, or a sudden sprain.

The main symptom is lower back pain on either or both sides, a pain that is lingering or off and on, which worsens when you are overexerted and lessens when you are relaxed. It can

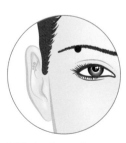

be a sharp stabbing pain, and it worsens when pressed. Lumbar spine hyperostosis, lumbar disc herniation, lumbar fractures, and tumors can all cause lower back pain. Diseases of the urinary system or reproductive system may also lead to lower back pain.

Mole in the eyebrow and nodules in the ear.

Face Reading

Those who have moles in the eyebrows

are prone to lower back pain. The bulge and deformity in the lumbosacral vertebrae zone of the ears turning to nodules is a warning sign of lumbar degeneration.

Therapeutic Methods

Make sure that you get plenty of rest during an onset of lower back pain, and some massage can be done to relieve the pain. Proper care in daily life can prevent the onset and alleviate the pain.

Dietary advice: Maintain a light diet, with plenty of vegetables, fruit, and beans. Consume foods that tone the lower back and kidney, promote blood circulation, and dredge collaterals, such as walnuts or Chinese wolfberries.

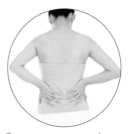

Some massage can be done to relieve the pain.

Exercise: Don't sit still for too long, instead, change your posture from time to time. Do some low intensity exercises, such as walking or yoga.

Lifestyle: Avoid staying in a humid environment, keep your lower back warm, and avoid catching colds. Avoid carrying heavy weights to protect the lower back from strain.

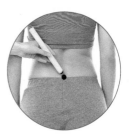

Yaoyangguan point.

Moxibustion: Perform moxibustion on the Weizhong point to relax tendons and alleviate pain, the Shenshu and Dachangshu points to invigorate the kidney and replenish essence to enhance *qi* and blood, and the Yaoyangguan point to relax tendons and sooth meridians, alleviating or eliminating pain. Gentle moxibustion at each of these acupoints for 15 minutes once daily can relieve lower back pain.

Massage: Massage the Weizhong point on the pathway of the Taiyang Bladder Meridian of the Foot. It has the

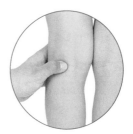

Weizhong point.

effect of relaxing the tendons and dredging collaterals, dispersing blood stasis and promoting blood circulation, clearing heat, and eliminating toxins. Press the Weizhong point with the tip of your thumb until a distension is felt, then press and release. This is considered one manipulation. Do this 10 to 20 times in a row. Massage once daily. Keep on massaging, and your lower back pain will be relieved.

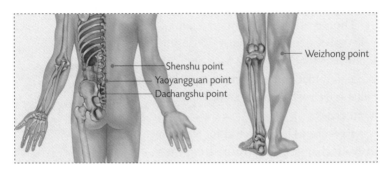

Shenshu point
Yaoyangguan point
Dachangshu point
Weizhong point

29. Frozen Shoulder

This is an inflammatory reaction caused by the degeneration of the shoulder joint capsule and surrounding soft tissue, common in people around 50 years old. It is more likely to affect women than men.

The clinical symptoms are shoulder pain, restricted shoulder movement, aversion to cold, pain when pressed, muscle cramps, and atrophy. The cause of the condition includes shoulder factors, such as the wear and tear of soft tissue in the elderly and long-term poor posture leading to chronic shoulder injuries. Cervical spondylosis and heart and lung diseases can also result in shoulder pain.

Face Reading

If skin pots or flaky redness appear in the shoulder zone of the ear, or white dots encircled by a tinge of redness at the edge, or perhaps turning dark red, these signs indicate inflammation of the shoulder joint or frozen shoulder.

Therapeutic Methods

In daily life, you can protect your shoulders by exercising more and taking supplementary calcium. At the onset of soreness and pain, massage or pat the shoulder gently for relief.

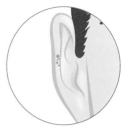

Flaky redness appear in the shoulder zone of the ear.

Dietary advice: To enhance nutrition intake, the middle-aged and elderly should pay special attention to the intake of supplementary calcium. Foods such as milk, eggs, soy products, bone soup, and fungus contain higher calcium.

Exercise: Do some shoulder exercises, such as pull-ups, patting the shoulders, shoulder shrugs, arm swings, and shoulder stretching.

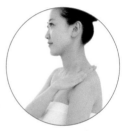

Massage or pat the shoulder gently for relief.

Lifestyle: Protect the shoulders from cold and wind, and avoid staying in humid places for too long. Standing and sitting postures should be correct. Avoid a sunken chest and hunchback, and avoid keeping your head down for too long in order to avoid stress to your neck and shoulders.

Moxibustion: Moxibustion at the Jianzhen, Jianliao, and Jianyu points can relax the tendons, activate the collaterals, and resolve stagnation. Moxibustion at the Shousanli and Bi'nao points can promote blood circulation and nourish the shoulders. Moxibustion with gentle warmth for 15 to 20 minutes at each acupoint once daily can relieve shoulder discomfort.

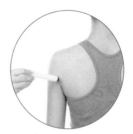

Jianzhen point.

Massage: Press the Hegu, Houxi, Shenmen, Daling, Taiyuan, Yemen, and Zhongchong points with your finger (any

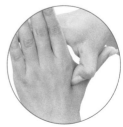

Hegu point.

finger) for one to three minutes, three to five times every day. When combined with shoulder exercises, this can promote blood circulation in the shoulders, thereby alleviating shoulder pain.

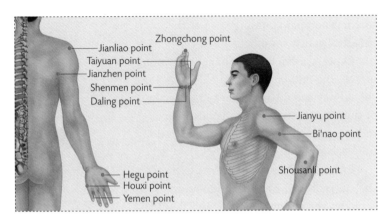

30. Irregular Menstruation

A common condition in gynecology, irregular menstruation refers to pathological changes in the menstrual cycle, with the volume of bleeding, color, and quality changing in the menstrual discharge. It is manifested as an abnormal menstrual cycle or volume of bleeding, which are often accompanied by abdominal pain and systemic symptoms before and during menstruation.

Irregular menstruation is clinically characterized as irregular menstrual cycles, too much or too little menstrual blood, abdominal pain, lower back pain, and even general body aches during the menstruation period. Factors such as cold attacks, irregular diet, and bad mood can all cause irregular menstruation. Weak kidney *qi*, stagnation of *qi* and blood, and deficiency of both *qi* and blood can also result in irregular menstruation.

Face Reading
The endocrine zone of women's ears shows dots or small dark red patches, and the kidney zone shows dots or small light

red patches. Women with irregular menstruation often have a dull yellow complexion.

Therapeutic Methods

If not treated in time, irregular menstruation can easily lead to other gynecological diseases, so much attention should be paid to this issue. Abdominal pain may occur during irregular menstruation.

Dietary advice: People with insufficient *qi* and blood can eat foods such as red dates and walnuts that have the properties of toning *qi* and blood. Those with stagnation of *qi* and blood stasis can eat foods such as haws and kelp that promote blood circulation and resolve blood stasis.

Exercise: During the non-menstrual period, do aerobic exercise that suit you, such as walking or jogging. These exercise will enhance your physical fitness and regulate the endocrine.

Emotional adjustment: Be relaxed both physically and mentally. Be happy, and avoid stress and mood swings. Maintain a peaceful state of mind, increase nutrition intake appropriately, and make sure you keep localized areas warm and clean during menstruation.

Medicinal diet therapy: Black bean soup. Wash 50 grams of black beans. Add water to the pot, then add the black beans. Bring it to the boil on high temperature, then simmer for about 10 minutes on low heat. Do not add too much water. When the bean soup is done, the darker the color, the better. It is good for

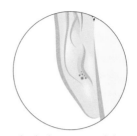

The kidney zone of the ear shows dots or small light red patches and a dull yellow complexion.

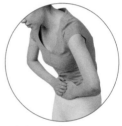

Abdominal pain may occur during irregular menstruation.

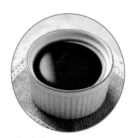

Black bean soup.

irregular menstruation caused by a kidney deficiency.

Moxibustion: Apply moxibustion to the Zhongji point to regulate menstruation and relieve pain. Apply to the Guanyuan point to nourish the kidney and replenish essence, to the Qihai point to enhance *yang* and replenish *qi*, and to the

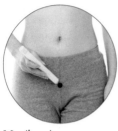

Sanyinjiao point to promote *qi* and blood transformation. Gentle moxibustion should be applied to these acupoints for 15 to 20 minutes per acupoint, once daily. This can relieve symptoms of irregular menstruation. Make sure that moxibustion is applied directly over the skin, unblocked.

Moxibustion.

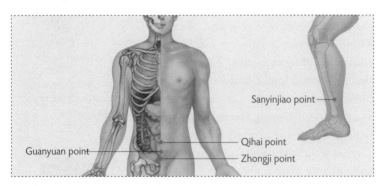

Sanyinjiao point

Guanyuan point

Qihai point

Zhongji point

31. Dysmenorrhea

Dysmenorrhea is classified into two types, primary and secondary. Primary dysmenorrhea is not an organic disease but recurrent menstrual pain, while secondary dysmenorrhea is caused by an organic disease of the pelvic cavity, such as endometriosis.

Dysmenorrhea is a condition characterized by recurrent abdominal cramps or distension during the menstrual cycle. Sometimes symptoms such as breast swelling, nausea, and cold limbs can also appear. Primary dysmenorrhea is a result of the obstruction of uterine blood flow leading to insufficient blood or oxygen supply to the muscle tissue of the uterus. Secondary dysmenorrhea is the result of a gynecological condition, tumors, or repeated early termination of a pregnancy.

Face Reading

Traditional Chinese medicine believes that dysmenorrhea results from cold and blood stasis in the body or a deficiency of blood and essence. Manifestations on the tongue include pale tongue with teeth impressions or cracks on the tongue, with little or no tongue coating, and there are petechiae on the edge or tip of the tongue, or stasis of collaterals on the underside of the tongue. In young women, telangiectasia in the triangular fossa zone of the ear, skin spots or small patches with a red tinge in the genital zone of the ear, or little dots with a red tinge on the endocrine zone of the ear.

Therapeutic Methods

Dysmenorrhea not only affects the patient's daily life but may also trigger other ailments. Measures should be taken to prevent and take care of it. During dysmenorrhea, drink warm water with brown sugar, which helps dispel cold to alleviate pain.

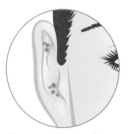

Skin spots or small patches with a red tinge in the ear.

Dietary advice: Avoid eating raw, cold, pungent, fatty, and greasy foods during menstruation. Avoid drinking strong tea, coffee, and liquor. A week before menstruation, you should have a diet that is light and nutritious.

Lifestyle: Make sure you stay warm during menstruation. You can put a hot water pouch at your lower abdomen and lower back to dispel cold and relieve pain. Rest during menstruation. Avoid taxing the mind, avoid severe stress, maintain

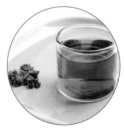

Warm water with brown sugar.

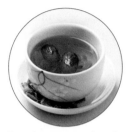

Dried orange peel and red dates tea.

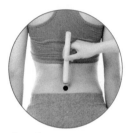

Shiqizhui point.

a peaceful state of mind, and avoid over exertion that can cause both physical and mental stress.

Medicinal diet therapy: Dried orange peel and red dates tea. Dried orange peel 5 g, two red dates. Wash the dried orange peel and red dates, put them in an earthenware pot, add water, and bring to the boil on high temperature, then simmer for 20 minutes on low heat. Drink it while it is warm. This tea is good for patients with dysmenorrhea because it works to invigorate *qi* and replenish the spleen, tone *qi*, and replenish blood. Add some ginger to the tea to dispel cold.

Moxibustion: For those with insufficient menstrual blood, apply moxibustion to the Guanyuan point to replenish essence and blood, to the Hegu and Sanyinjiao points to promote *qi* and blood, promote blood circulation, and relieve pain, and to the Shiqizhui point to relax muscles and clear collaterals, soothe menstruation, and alleviate pain. Apply mild-warm moxibustion to these points, for about 15 minutes each, once daily.

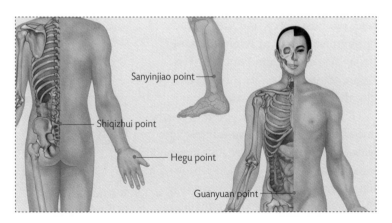

Sanyinjiao point

Shiqizhui point

Hegu point

Guanyuan point

32. Hyperplasia of the Breast

Hyperplasia refers to an overgrowth of epithelium and fibrous tissue in the breast, the structural degeneration of breast tissue ducts and lobules, and the overgrowth of progressive connective tissue. Hyperplasia of the breast is a common condition in women.

Hyperplasia is characterized by recurrent pain in the breasts, which is aggravated before menstruation each month and is relieved or disappears after menstruation. In severe cases, the pain persists before and after menstruation. Hyperplasia is a result of endocrine dysfunction. Psychological factors, such as a bad mood and irritability, are also pathogenic factors.

Face Reading

TCM teaches that hyperplasia of the breast is mainly caused by stagnation of liver *qi* and emotional factors. The tongue will exhibit a pale texture with a white coating, or reddish texture with dry coating. At the same time, the corresponding reflex zone on the face will show nodules or white spots. In women, there are fleshy bumps in the inner canthus. White spots are shown on their thoracic vertebrae zone of the ears, and they will speak with their heads and mouths tilted to one side. All of the above suggest breast hyperplasia.

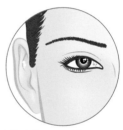

Nodules or white spots in the ear, and fleshy bumps in the inner canthus.

Therapeutic Methods

In addition to treatment with drugs, therapies for hyperplasia should start with the diet, lifestyle, exercise, and mood. Frequent rubbing of the breasts can dredge the ducts to relieve breast pain.

Dietary advice: The overall diet should be low in fat and rich in vitamins. Maintain

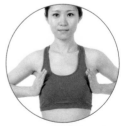

Frequent rubbing of the breasts can dredge the ducts to relieve breast pain.

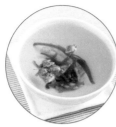

Rose flower and kelp soup.

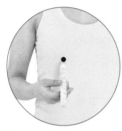

Rugen point.

a balanced diet to prevent obesity.

Exercise: Continue to engage in physical exercise, but focus mainly on aerobic exercise. Do not engage in strenuous activity. Chest expansion exercises can help relieve pain.

Emotional adjustment: Learn to control your mood, resolve negative emotions promptly, and avoid being sulky or indulging in long-term depression, worry, and sadness, so as to prevent aggravating the pain.

Medicinal diet therapy: Rose flower and kelp soup. Rose flowers 15 g, kelp 100 g, dried orange peel 5 g. Wash the kelp and shred it. Wash the dried orange peels and tear them into strips. Put the rose flowers, kelp, and orange peel in an earthenware pot and cook for 40 minutes over low heat. This decoction is suitable for patients with hyperplasia caused by liver depression and phlegm stagnation. Rose flowers are effective for promoting blood circulation and removing stasis.

Moxibustion: Apply to the Rugen, Zhongfu, and Danzhong points to sooth the chest and regulate *qi* to relieve breast pain, and to the Zusanli, Fenglong, and Sanyinjiao points to promote blood circulation and relieve pain. Apply mild-warm moxibustion at the acupoints above for 15 minutes each, once daily.

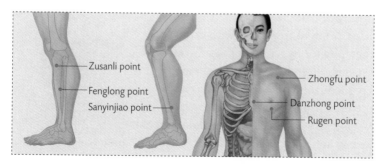

33. Uterine Fibroids

Uterine fibroids are benign tumors in the female genitalia that are manifested as an enlarged uterus and in abnormal menstruation. Uterine fibroids are composed of smooth muscle and connective tissue. The condition is more common in middle-aged women.

Clinically, the main symptom of uterine fibroids is masses, which may lead to uterine bleeding, abdominal fullness or pain, abnormal leucorrhea, anemia, infertility, and miscarriages. Western medicine believes that uterine fibroids may be related to long-term high levels of estrogen in the body, whereas TCM holds that uterine fibroids are related to coagulated cold in uterus, stagnation of *qi* and blood stasis, and dysfunction of the spleen's transportation.

Face Reading

Women who have dark hooked or spiral blood vessels in the outer canthal triangle of the eye are prone to uterine fibroids. Women with one or multiple dark red blood vessels under the outer corner of the eye may have uterine fibroids.

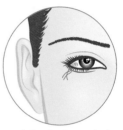

Dark hooked or spiral blood vessels in the outer canthal triangle of the eye and dark red blood vessels under the outer corner of the eye.

Therapeutic Methods

Uterine fibroids are not easy to detect, so diligent observation is required. Watch out for any abnormalities and go to the doctor for checkups. In daily life you can take some preventive measures. Frequently pressing and kneading the lower abdomen can promote blood circulation, resolve stasis, and alleviate symptoms of fibroids.

Dietary advice: Consume a light diet. It is not advisable to eat foods such as chicken and crabs, which may trigger the disease. Be cautious with foods or health

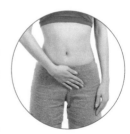

Frequently pressing and kneading the lower abdomen can promote blood circulation.

products that contain estrogen.

Exercise: Patients with uterine fibroids should be actively engaged in exercise to improve their physical fitness. Aerobic exercise such as running, swimming, and yoga are good options.

Emotional adjustment: Avoid losing your temper during menstruation, which can lead to stagnation of *qi* and leave you prone to uterine fibroids. It is important to be relaxed and positive to prevent the formation of fibroids.

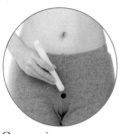

Moxibustion: Apply to the Qugu, Guanyuan, Zigong, and Sanyinjiao to invigorate *qi* and promote blood circulation, eliminate phlegm, and resolve blood stasis. Apply mild-warm moxibustion to these acupoints, once daily, 15 minutes each time, until a warm and comfortable sensation is produced on the skin.

Qugu point.

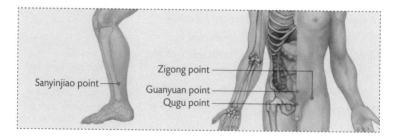

34. Ovarian Cysts

Ovarian cysts are a common gynecological condition most common in women aged between 20 and 50.

The clinical manifestation of ovarian cysts is that they are mobile, consisting of medium-sized sacs or pockets in the abdomen that generally present no discomfort or pain and can often move from the pelvic cavity to the abdominal cavity. The pathogenesis of ovarian cysts is relatively complex, and multiple factors are to blame, including genetics, environment, hormones, viruses, and other factors. Among them, environment and hormones are the two leading pathogenic factors.

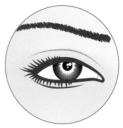

Face Reading
The patient's pupils are significantly reduced, suggesting ovarian cysts.

The patient's pupils are significantly reduced.

Therapeutic Methods
Ovarian cysts are mostly benign in the early stage. If not treated in a timely manner and allowed to develop, they may deteriorate. Preventive measures should be taken in one's daily life. Patients should not eat foods containing hormones, such as royal jelly.

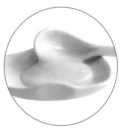

Patients should not eat foods containing hormones, such as royal jelly.

Dietary advice: Consume a light diet, avoid pungent foods or foods and health products that contain estrogen, and take vitamins and calcium.

Exercise: Engage in physical exercise to enhance your physical fitness. Regulate your hormone balance and maintain a normal secretion of hormones in the body to prevent ovarian cysts.

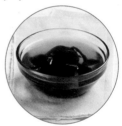

Emotional adjustment: Relax and avoid being angry. Cysts that are less than five centimeters in diameter will gradually shrink or even disappear. Don't be anxious about the condition.

Brown sugar soup with haws and fungus.

Medicinal diet therapy: Brown sugar soup with haws and fungus. Haws 50 g, fungus 30 g, and brown sugar. Decoct the haws in about 500 ml of water, then remove the residue, but keep the soup. Add the soaked fungus and simmer on low heat until well-done. Finally, add brown sugar and mix well. This soup, which promotes blood circulation and removes blood stasis, is suitable for patients with irregular menstruation caused

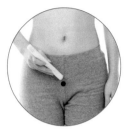

Zhongji point.

by ovarian cysts.

Moxibustion: The principal acupoints: ① the Qugu point for regulating menstruation and alleviating pain, ② the Zhongji point for strengthening the middle burner and replenishing *qi*, ③ the Guanyuan point for regulating the meridian and clearing the lower burner, and ④ the Guilai point for warming the meridian and dispelling cold, promoting blood circulation, and resolving stasis. The principal points are treated every day, once daily for 15 minutes. The auxiliary acupoints, the Xingjian, Qimen, Zhongfeng, and Qihai, can be treated in turn every day. Use the pad of your thumb to press-knead the auxiliary points once or twice daily, for three to five minutes each. Frequent moxibustion of these points can effectively relieve the symptoms of ovarian cysts.

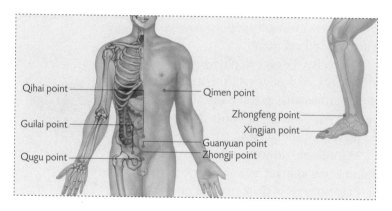

35. Infertility

Women in their reproductive years who have no fertility problems and have normal sex lives and are not using contraceptives, but have not been able to conceive after having been sexually active for a year, or those who were previously impregnated but have not become pregnant after discontinuing the use of contraceptives for more than one year are considered infertile.

Infertility is clinically manifested as failure to get pregnant over a long period. The condition can also be accompanied by symptoms such as irregular menstruation, lower abdominal pain, lumbosacral pain, and abnormal leucorrhea. Modern medicine classifies the causes of infertility into five categories: ovulation dysfunctions, fallopian tube obstructions, underdeveloped uterus, chronic cervicitis or pelvic inflammatory disease, and congenital malformations that affect one's sex life.

Face Reading
If a woman's philtrum is flat or almost invisible, this indicates infertility. If the width of the philtrum is almost the same from top to bottom and the edges on both sides of the groove are evidently thicker, this suggests congenital infertility.

Therapeutic Methods
Infertility is caused by both internal and external factors, so patients with infertility need internal regulation and external nourishment in order to improve. They should go to the hospital for an examination when they have concerns about pregnancy, and they would follow the doctor's advice for treatment.

Dietary advice: Balance your nutritional intake, and make sure that you have sufficient intake of essential proteins, vitamins, and micro-elements, which provide sufficient nutrition for ovulation.

Exercise: Do more low intensity and relaxing exercise, such as yoga or walking. These exercise can not only strengthen your body and improve your immunity, but also relax your mood.

Emotional adjustment: Adjust your state of mind and keep your mood balanced. In many cases, the eagerness for a child will only further interfere with

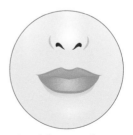

The philtrum is flat or almost invisible.

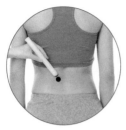

Shenshu point.

endocrine function, making it difficult to conceive.

Moxibustion: Apply to the Shenshu point as the main point, which has the effect of invigorating kidney *qi*, and combined with the Yaoyangguan and Zhongji points, which can improve the deficiency of *qi* and blood. Or apply to the Taichong point as the main point, which has the effect of dispelling phlegm and clearing blood stasis, and when combined with the Sanyinjiao point, it can invigorate the spleen, sooth the liver, and tone the kidney. The main acupoints are generally treated every day, but the auxiliary acupoints can be treated in rotation for 15 minutes each, once daily. Moxibustion of these acupoints can strengthen the functions of the liver, spleen, and kidneys to enhance the patient's ability to conceive.

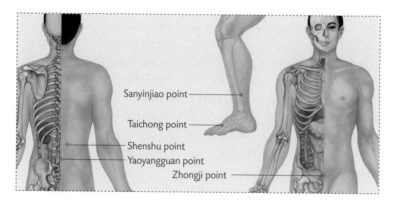

Sanyinjiao point
Taichong point
Shenshu point
Yaoyangguan point
Zhongji point

36. Chronic Prostatitis

A chronic inflammation of the prostate gland caused by various factors, chronic prostatitis is a common disease in urology that includes chronic bacterial prostatitis and non-bacterial prostatitis.

The clinical symptoms of chronic prostatitis are prostate

pain, frequent urination, an urgent need to urinate, pain when urinating, a burning urethra, and cloudy urine, which may be accompanied by dizziness, tinnitus, insomnia, dreamy nights, anxiety and depression, and even impotence and premature ejaculation. The causes of this condition include prostate congestion, urine irritation, pathogenic microorganism infection, anxiety, and depression.

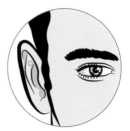

Curved blood vessels in the eye and small nodules in the ear.

Face Reading

Deep curved blood vessels in the outer canthal triangle area of the eye and small nodules in the angle of superior concha zone of the ear suggest chronic prostatitis.

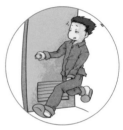

Therapeutic Methods

Symptoms of mild chronic prostatitis can be relieved through daily care.

The clinical symptoms include frequent urination, an urgent need to urinate and pain when urinating.

Dietary advice: Consume a light diet, avoid pungent and highly acidic foods, and don't drink liquor. Eat plenty of fruits, vegetables, and seeds.

Exercise: Do exercises with your anus. Tighten the sphincter muscle and pull it up, then relax. Do this repeatedly to promote the circulation of *qi* and blood in the prostate to alleviate inflammation.

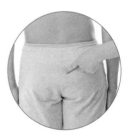

Huiyang point.

Emotional adjustment: Patients should maintain a balanced state of mind, understand the condition of chronic prostatitis, and avoid excessive worry. Maintain a positive mood, develop a positive attitude toward the treatment, and actively cooperate in it.

Massage: The Huiyang point dissipates water and dampness, replenishes *yang*, and nourishes *qi*. Curve your fingers to loosely

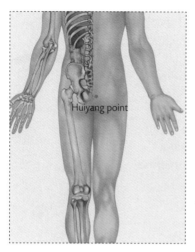

form a hollowed fist with both
hands, use the prominent joints
of the thumb to knead-press
the Huiyang point with both
hands at the same time. Apply
enough force to make the
acupoint feel the distension.
Do this twice a day for five
minutes each time. Massaging
this point often has good
effects on diarrhea, bloody
stool, hemorrhoids, impotence,
and prostatitis.

37. Erectile Dysfunction

Erectile dysfunction refers to the condition in which a man not
yet reaching the age of sexual decline has sexual desires, but is
unable to have an erection, or the erection is not firm enough or
does not last long enough to have successful intercourse.

Patients often have accompanying symptoms such as a pale
complexion, anxiety, panic, weariness and fatigue, weakness in
the lower back and knees, aversion to cold and cold limbs, or
difficulty urinating and low urine output. The causes of erectile
dysfunction are mainly related to factors such as excessive sex,
worry and fear, anxiety and irritability, long-term inflammation
of the urinary system, and stagnation of the liver *qi*.

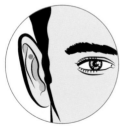

Face Reading
When the internal and external genitalia
zones of the ear show flaking or grayish-
white spots, this can be a sign of erectile
dysfunction.

Grayish-white spots in
the ear.

Therapeutic Methods
Erectile dysfunction is a common

condition in men. Measures can be taken to prevent it, and therapeutic treatments can be effective in several aspects.

Dietary advice: Many patients tend to have deficiency syndromes. They should maintain proper supplementary nutrition intake and eat foods that have warming and invigorating effects, such as lamb, beef, red dates, and walnuts, and avoid raw and cold foods, as well as those foods that have a cold property.

Exercise: Increase physical exercise, as exercise can promote the circulation of *qi* and blood. Choose exercise suited to your own situation, e.g. long-distance running, swimming, and ball games.

Emotional adjustment: Maintain an optimistic attitude, abstain from masturbation, balance work and rest, participate in more recreational activities, be cheerful, and maintain a harmonious relationship with your spouse.

Medicinal diet therapy: Lamb soup cooked with Chinese wolfberries and Chinese yam. Lamb 250 g, Chinese yam 50 g, some Chinese wolfberries, salt, and ginger slices. Wash the lamb and slice it, then blanch to remove the blood from the lamb. Peel the Chinese yam and wash it, then dice and score it. Put all the ingredients into a pot and cook until very tender, then add salt to taste. This soup can tone deficiencies, dispel cold, warm the kidneys, and replenish *yang*.

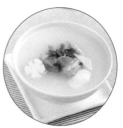

Lamb soup cooked with Chinese wolfberries and Chinese yam.

Massage: Massage the Yaoyangguan point, where the kidney *yin* and the kidney *yang* of the human body intersect and which can replenish kidney *qi* and invigorate essence and blood, thereby toning both *yin* and *yang*. Use your thumb to massage the Yaoyangguan point in a rotating manner. Press-knead 50 to 100

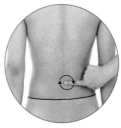

Yaoyangguan point.

times each session, once or twice daily, for about three to five minutes. This has a good effect on men having problems with the reproductive system, such as erectile dysfunction, helping to relieve and prevent conditions of the male reproductive system.

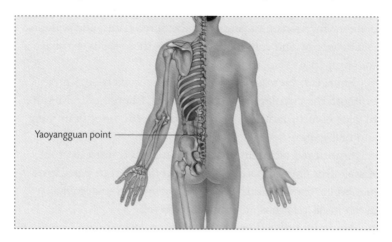

Yaoyangguan point

38. Nocturnal Emissions

Nocturnal emissions are a result of a deficiency of the spleen and kidney, leading to the functional failure to hold the fluid, or of damp-heat disturbing the essence chamber. Frequent leaking of semen unrelated to sexual activity is considered an ailment.

Clinically, nocturnal emissions are manifested more than twice a week, often accompanied by such symptoms as lightheadedness, tinnitus, forgetfulness, palpitations and anxiety, insomnia, and dreaminess. Some patients can also display other symptoms such as frequent urination, an urgency to urinate, and painful urination. The condition can be caused by unrestrained sexual activity, a congenital deficiency, over-thinking, unfulfilled desires, unhealthy eating habits, and an attack of damp-heat.

Face Reading
If oily, moist red patches appear in the triangular fossa zone of

the ear, it suggests that frequent nocturnal emissions have caused fatigue and lower back pain.

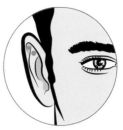

Oily, moist red patches appear in the triangular fossa zone of the ear.

Therapeutic Methods

Patients should learn to adjust their state of mind and know how not to be a captive of sexual desire, and to instead cultivate the mind. At the same time restraint should be exercised in sex activity and masturbation should be avoided.

Dietary advice: This condition is mostly a result of a deficiency syndrome. Patients should maintain a diet focused on nourishment and avoid foods that are raw, cold, or of a cold property. Those with hyperactivity of fire due to *yin* deficiency should avoid foods that are dry and of a warm property. Those with unconsolidated kidney *qi* should eat walnuts, black beans, and similar foods.

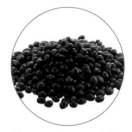

Those with unconsolidated kidney *qi* should eat walnuts, black beans, and similar foods.

Exercise: Persevere in the engagement of physical activities of appropriate intensity, such as walking, jogging, ball games, or yoga, but avoid over-exertion.

Emotional adjustment: Focus on mental adjustment and cultivation, keep away from unnecessary arousal, and lead a life of few desires. Cultivate a peaceful mind and hobbies to enrich your life, and avoid over-exertion.

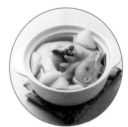

Chicken stewed with Chinese yam and Chinese wolfberries.

Medicinal diet therapy: Chicken stewed with Chinese yam and Chinese wolfberries. Chinese yam 500 g, one chicken, Chinese wolfberries, and salt. Wash the chicken and cut into pieces, add some water, and cook on high heat until it is half done. Wash the Chinese yam, peel the skin, and cut it into pieces. Put it into the pot, then add the Chinese wolfberries and salt and cook until squashy. Regular intake of this medicinal dish can nourish the kidney and strengthen the essence.

Massage: The Shenmen point calms the nerves, tranquilizes the mind, and clears the meridians. It is mainly used to treat

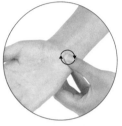

heart palpitations, insomnia, and forgetfulness. Combined with the Taixi and Zusanli points, it can alleviate, to some extent, symptoms resulting from nocturnal emission, such as heart palpitations and insomnia. Massage once or twice a day for three to five minutes each using the pad of your thumb.

Shenmen point.

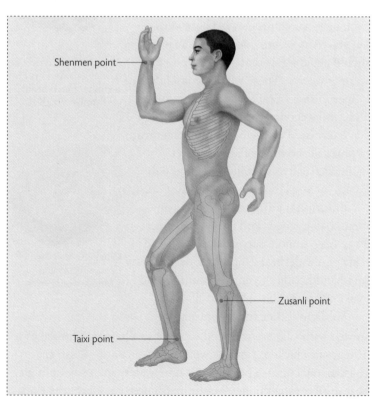

Appendices

Body Inch Measurements

1. Using Thumb Length	2. Using Middle-Finger Length	3. Using Four Fingers Closed Together
The width of the patient's thumb joint is 1 body inch. This is applicable for locating the acupoint on four limbs with vertical body inches.	With the patient's middle sections of the bent middle finger as measurement, the distance between two inner crease tips is taken as 1 body inch, which is mostly applicable for locating acupoints on the four limbs and the back.	With the index finger, middle finger, ring finger, and small finger stretched straight and closed, measure at the level of the large knuckle (the second joint) of the middle finger. The width of the four fingers is 3 body inches.

1 body inch

1 body inch

3 body inches

Location of Acupoints

Acupoint	Code	Location	Fast Localization
Baihui	GV 20	On the head, 5 body inches superior to the anterior hairline, on the anterior midline.	When seated, in the depression at the crossing point of the arch connecting the ear apex and the midline on the head.
Bailao	EX-HN 15	On the neck, 2 body inches straight superior to the seventh cervical spine, and 1 body inch lateral to the middle line of the back.	In a prone or sitting position, 2 body inches directly and one finger's breadth lateral above Dazhui point (GV 14).
Bi'nao	LI 14	On the lateral aspect of the arm, just anterior to the border of the deltoid muscle, 7 body inches superior to Quchi point (LI 11).	With elbow flexed and the deltoid muscle bulged while forming a fist, the point is on the inferior portion of the deltoid of the medial side, feeling soreness and distention on palpation.
Chengqi	ST 1	On the face, between the eye and the infraorbital margin, directly inferior to the pupil.	With index finger and middle finger straight and close together, put the tip of the middle finger on the lateral side of the nose. The point is under the infraorbital rim at the point the tip of the index finger touches.
Chize	LU 5	On the anterior aspect of the elbow, at the cubital crease, in the depression lateral to the biceps brachii tendon.	Elbow flexed, on the lateral border of the tendon.

Acupoint	Code	Location	Fast Localization
Dachangshu	BL 25	In the lumbar region, at the same level as the inferior border of the spinous process of the fourth lumbar vertebra, 1.5 body inches lateral to the posterior midline.	Refer to the location.
Daheng	SP 15	On the upper abdomen, 4 body inches lateral to the center of the umbilicus.	4 body inches lateral to the umbilicus.
Daling	PC 7	On the anterior aspect of the wrist, between the tendons of palmaris longus and the flexor carpi radialis, on the palmar wrist crease.	Wrist flexed slightly and fist made, the midpoint of the first transverse crease of wrist and between two tendons.
Danzhong	CV 17	In the anterior thoracic region, at the same level as the fourth intercostal space, on the anterior midline.	On the chest, at the level of the fourth intercostals, on the anterior midline (between the nipples).
Dazhu	BL 11	In the upper back region, at the same level as the inferior border of the spinous process of the first thoracic vertebra, 1.5 body inches lateral to the posterior midline.	With neck flexed, 1.5 body inches breadth lateral to the lower border of the vertebra one down from the top.
Dazhui	GV 14	In the posterior region of the neck, in the depression inferior to the spinous process of the seventh cervical vertebra, on the posterior midline.	With head lowered, in the depression of the lower border of the biggest vertebra of the neck.

Acupoint	Code	Location	Fast Localization
Dubi	ST 35	On the anterior aspect of the knee, in the depression lateral to the patellar ligament.	In a sitting position, extending the lower limbs forcefully and straightly, in the depression on the inferior lateral border of the knee.
Feishu	BL 13	In the upper back region, at the same level as the inferior border of the spinous process of the third thoracic vertebra, 1.5 body inches lateral to the posterior midline.	With neck flexed, 1.5 body inches breadth lateral to the lower border of the vertebra three down from the top vertebra.
Fengchi	GB 20	In the posterior region of the neck, inferior to the occipital bone, in the depression between the origins of sternocleidomastoid and the trapezius muscles.	In a sitting position, in the depression on the lateral border of the two tendons on the back of head, at the level of earlobe.
Fenglong	ST 40	On the anterolateral aspect of the leg, lateral border of the tibialis anterior muscle, 8 body inches superior to the prominence of the external malleolus.	In a sitting position, knee flexed, at the midpoint of the line from Dubi point (ST 35) to the tip of the external malleolus, 1.5 body inches width to the tibial crest.
Guanyuan	CV 4	On the lower abdomen, 3 body inches inferior to the center of the umbilicus, on the anterior midline.	On the lower abdomen, four fingers' breadth directly below the umbilicus, on the anterior midline.
Guilai	ST 29	On the lower abdomen, 4 body inches inferior to the center of the umbilicus, 2 body inches lateral to anterior midline.	In a supine position, one finger's breadth above the upper border of symphysis pubis, 2 body inches lateral to the anterior midline.

Acupoint	Code	Location	Fast Localization
Hegu	LI 4	On the dorsum of the hand, radial to the midpoint of the second metacarpal bone.	Closing the index finger and thumb, on the top of the muscle.
Houxi	SI 3	On the dorsum of the hand, in the depression proximal to the ulnar side of the fifth metacarpophalangeal joint, at the border between the red and white flesh.	Forming a fist, on the posterior border of the fifth metacarpophalangeal joint, at the border between the red and white flesh.
Huagai	CV 20	In the anterior thoracic region, at the same level as the first intercostal space, on the anterior midline.	On the chest, at the level of the first intercostals, on the anterior midline.
Huiyang	BL 35	In the sacral region, 0.5 body inches lateral to the extremity of the coccyx.	In a prone position, 0.5 body inches lateral to the end of the spine.
Jianjing	GB 21	At the midpoint of the line connecting the spinous process of the seventh cervical vertebra with the lateral end of the acromion.	The midpoint between Yangbai point (GB 14) and acromial end of the clavicle.
Jianliao	TE 14	On the shoulder girdle, in the depression between the acromial angle and the greater tubercle of the humerus.	Refer to the location.
Jianyu	LI 15	On the shoulder girdle, in the depression between the anterior end of the lateral border of the acromion and the greater tubercle of the humerus.	Seated straight, flex the elbow and raise the arm as high as the shoulder. The point is in the depression present on the shoulder when the middle finger presses the shoulder tip.

Acupoint	Code	Location	Fast Localization
Jianzhen	SI 9	On the shoulder girdle, posteroinferior to the shoulder joint, 1 body inch superior to the posterior axillary fold.	In a sitting position with shoulder relaxed, one finger's breadth above the end of the posterior axillary fold.
Cervical Jiaji	EX-B 2 (Jiaji)	On both sides of the middle line of the neck, 0.5 body inches away from the lower edge of the spinous process of the first to seventh cervical vertebra, with seven points each side.	Refer to the location.
Jingqu	LU 8	On the anterolateral aspect of the forearm, between the radial styloid process and the radial artery, 1 body inch superior to the palmar wrist crease.	With palm up, between the radial styloid process and the radial artery, one finger's breadth superior to the palmar wrist crease.
Kongzui	LU 6	On the anterolateral aspect of the forearm, on the line connecting Chize point (LU 5) with Taiyuan point (LU 9), 7 body inches superior to the palmar wrist crease.	With arm extended forward with palm up, on the line from Chize point (LU 5) and Taiyuan point (LU 9), one finger's breadth superior to the midpoint.
Neiguan	PC 6	On the anterior aspect of the forearm, between the tendons of the palmaris longus and the flexor carpi radialis, 2 body inches proximal to the palmar wrist crease.	Wrist flexed slightly and fist made, 2 body inches above the transverse crease of the wrist and between the two tendons.
Neiting	ST 44	On the dorsum of the foot, between the second and third toes, posterior to the web margin, at the border between the red and white flesh.	On the dorsum of the foot, between the second and third toes, at the junction of the red and white flesh.

Acupoint	Code	Location	Fast Localization
Pishu	BL 20	In the upper back region, at the same level as the inferior border of the spinous process of the 11th thoracic vertebra, 1.5 body inches lateral to the posterior midline.	1.5 body inches lateral to the lower border of that three more vertebras up from the vertebra at the level of the umbilicus.
Qihai	CV 6	On the lower abdomen, 1.5 body inches inferior to the center of the umbilicus, on the anterior midline.	On the lower abdomen, 1.5 body inches directly below the umbilicus, on the anterior midline.
Qimen	LR 14	In the anterior thoracic region, in the sixth intercostal space, 4 body inches lateral to the anterior midline.	While sitting or lying on one side, in the second intercostal space directly below the nipple, feeling soreness and distention on pressure.
Qingling	HT 2	On the medial aspect of the arm, just medial to the biceps brachii muscle, 3 body inches superior to the cubital crease.	Arm extending, on the line between Shaohai point (HT 3) and Jiquan point (HT 1), 4 fingers' breadth above Shaohai point (HT 3).
Quchi	LI 11	On the lateral aspect of the elbow, at the midpoint of the line connecting Chize point (LU 5) with the lateral epicondyle of the humerus.	Arm flexed, at the end to the transverse cubital crease, close to the tip of elbow.
Qugu	CV 2	On the lower abdomen, superior to the pubic symphysis, on the anterior midline.	On the upper border of the bone landmark transversely distributed in the lower abdomen, on the anterior midline.

Acupoint	Code	Location	Fast Localization
Rugen	ST 18	In the anterior thoracic region, in the fifth intercostal space, 4 body inches lateral to the anterior midline.	Refer to the location.
Sanyinjiao	SP 6	On the tibial aspect of the leg, posterior to the medial border of the tibia, 3 body inches superior to the prominence of the medial malleolus.	In a sitting or supine position, posterior to the medial border of the tibia, four fingers' breadth directly above the tip of the medial malleolus.
Shangqu	KI 17	On the upper abdomen, 2 body inches superior to the center of the umbilicus, 0.5 body inches lateral to the anterior midline.	In a supine position, 2 body inches above the umbilicus, 0.5 body inches lateral.
Shaochong	HT 9	On the little finger, radial to the distal phalanx, 0.1 body inches proximal-lateral to the radial corner of the little fingernail, at the intersection of the vertical line of the radial border of the nail and horizontal line of the base of the little fingernail.	The little finger extending, at the crossing point of the line along the transverse line of the lower nail border and the longitudinal line on the radial side of the nail.
Shenmen	HT 7	On the anteromedial aspect of the wrist, radial to the flexor carpi ulnaris tendon, on the palmar wrist crease.	Loosely making a fist, hold the wrist with the hand and the thumb flexed. The point is in the depression where the nail touches the hand.

Acupoint	Code	Location	Fast Localization
Shenshu	BL 23	In the lumbar region, at the same level as the inferior border of the spinous process of the second lumbar vertebra, 1.5 body inches lateral to the posterior midline.	1.5 body inches breadth lateral to the lower border of the vertebra at the level of the umbilicus.
Shenzhu	GV 12	In the upper back region, in the depression inferior to the spinous process of the third thoracic vertebra, on the posterior midline.	In the depression of the lower border of that four vertebras up from the one at the level of the line between the inferior scaplular angles, on the posterior midline.
Shiqizhui	EX-B 8	On the waist, and on the middle line of the back, the depression under the fifth lumbar spine.	One vertebra down from the one passing the line of bilateral iliac spines, inferior to the spinous process.
Shousanli	LI 10	On the posterolateral aspect of the forearm, on the line connecting Yangxi point (LI 5) with Quchi point (LI 11), 2 body inches inferior to the cubital crease.	Elbow flexed, 2 body inches inferior to the end of the transverse cubital crease.
Shuaigu	GB 8	On the head, directly superior to the auricular apex, 1.5 body inches superior to the temporal hairline.	Directly above the ear apex, 1.5 body inches breadth within the hairline.
Taichong	LR 3	On the dorsum of the foot, between the first and second metatarsal bones, in the depression distal to the junction of the bases of the two bones, over the dorsalis pedis artery.	On the dorsum of the foot, in the depression on between the first and second metatarsal bones.

Acupoint	Code	Location	Fast Localization
Taixi	KI 3	On the posteromedial aspect of the ankle, in the depression between the prominence of the medial malleolus and the calcaneal tendon.	In a sitting position, in the depression between the medial malleolus and the Achilles tendon.
Taiyang	EX-HN 5	On the temporal, between the tip of the brow and outer canthal, the depression that 1 body inch behind and inferior to it.	In a sitting or supine position, in the depression lateral to the outer end of eyebrow.
Taiyuan	LU 9	On the anterolateral aspect of the wrist, between the radial styloid process and the scaphoid bone, in the depression ulnar to the abductor pollicis longus tendon.	Palm up, on the lateral side of the radial artery lateral to the wrist crease.
Weizhong	BL 40	On the posterior aspect of the knee, at the midpoint of the popliteal crease.	On the back of knee, in the center of the popliteal crease.
Xinshu	BL 15	In the upper back region, at the same level as the inferior border of the spinous process of the fifth thoracic vertebra, 1.5 body inches lateral to the posterior midline.	1.5 body inches breadth lateral to the lower border of the two vertebras up from the vertebra at the level of the inferior scapular angle.
Xiyan	EX-LE 5	When the knee is flexed, the point is in the depression medial to the patellar ligament. The point on the inner side is called Neixiyan (inner Xiyan) while the point on the outer side is called Waixiyan (outer Xiyan).	Refer to the location.

Acupoint	Code	Location	Fast Localization
Yanglingquan	GB 34	On the fibular aspect of the leg, in the depression anterior and distal to the head of the fibula.	Bend knee flexed at 90°, on the lateral and inferior of the knee joint, in the depression anterior and inferior to the small head of the fibula.
Yaoyangguan	GV 3	In the lumbar region, in the depression inferior to the spinous process of the fourth lumbar vertebra, on the posterior midline.	In a prone position, in the depression at the level of the spinous process of the uppermost ends of the hip joints.
Yemen	TE 2	On the dorsum of the hand, in the depression superior to the web margin between the ring and little fingers, at the border between the red and white skin.	With a loosely held fist and palm down, on the web of the fourth and fifth fingers, at the junction between red and white skin.
Yingxiang	LI 20	On the face, in the nasolabial sulcus, at the same level as the midpoint of lateral border of the ala of the nose.	In the depression lateral to the nostril.
Yongquan	KI 1	On the sole of the foot, in the deepest depression when the foot is in plantar flexion.	Foot flexed, in the depression on the anterior 1/3 on the sole.
Zhongchong	PC 9	On the middle finger, at the center of the tip of the finger.	Palm down, in the center on the tip of middle finger.
Zhongfu	LU 1	On the anterior thoracic region, at the same level as the first intercostal space, lateral to the infraclavicular fossa, 6 body inches lateral to the anterior median line.	In a standing position, hands on the hips, one finger width below the depression inferior to the lateral side of the clavicle.

Acupoint	Code	Location	Fast Localization
Zhongji	CV 3	On the lower abdomen, 4 body inches inferior to the center of the umbilicus, on the anterior midline.	On the lower abdomen, one finger's breadth above Qugu point (CV 2), on the anterior midline.
Zhongwan	CV 12	On the upper abdomen, 4 body inches superior to the center of the umbilicus, on the anterior midline.	In supine, on the anterior midline, at the midpoint between the xiphisternal horn and the umbilicus.
Zigong	EX-CA 1	On the lower abdomen, 4 body inches inferior to the umbilical, and 3 body inches lateral to anterior midline.	Refer to the location.
Zusanli	ST 36	On the anterior aspect of the leg, on the line connecting Dubi point (ST 35) with Jiexi point (ST 41), 3 body inches inferior to Dubi point (ST 35) .	In a standing position, bend the body, match the web of the first and second interphalangeal fingers with the upper lateral border of the hand, place the rest fingers naturally downward, the point is where the tip of the middle finger touches.